# REAL FOOD FERMENTATION

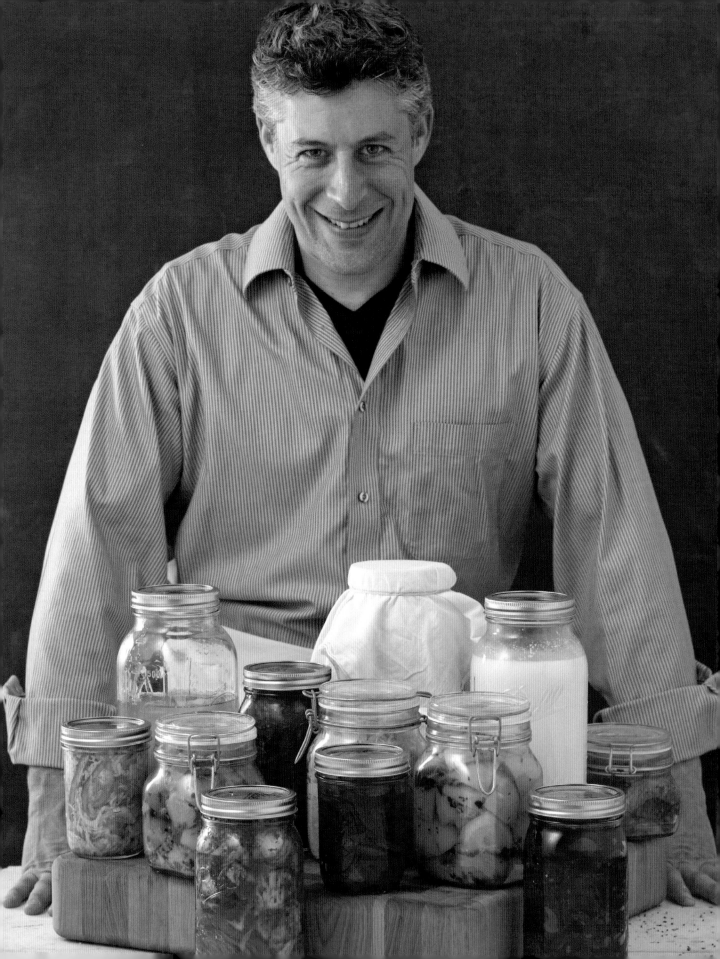

# REAL FOOD FERMENTATION

## Preserving Whole Fresh Food with Live Cultures in Your Home Kitchen

### ALEX LEWIN

**Quarry Books**
100 Cummings Center, Suite 406L
Beverly, MA 01915

quarrybooks.com • craftside.typepad.com

First published in the United States of America in 2012 by
Quarry Books, a member of
Quayside Publishing Group
100 Cummings Center
Suite 406-L
Beverly, Massachusetts 01915-6101
Telephone: (978) 282-9590
Fax: (978) 283-2742
www.quarrybooks.com

10 9 8 7 6 5

ISBN: 978-1-59253-784-6

Digital edition published in 2012
eISBN: 978-1-61058-417-3

Library of Congress Cataloging-in-Publication Data

Lewin, Alex.
Real food fermentation : preserving whole fresh food with live cultures in your home kitchen /
Alex Lewin. -- Digital ed.
    p. cm.
Summary: "Learn how to choose and prepare only the best, freshest ingredients for all your
kitchen fermenting projects with Real Food Fermentation!* Learn how to make tasty foods
including kimchi, yogurt, and sauerkraut* Improves digestion* Enzyme-rich foods contain
high nutrient value* Boosts "good" bacteria production. Fermentation is one of the earliest
forms of natural food preservation, and without it, our beloved vegetables, fruits, grains,
and milk would be heaps of moldy abundance after the harvest. Learn how to turn simple
ingredients into health goldmines such as kimchi, sauerkraut, kefir, kombucha, and more in
this flavorful book. Author and health strategist Alex Lewin empowers you with the tools,
techniques, instructions, and delicious recipes to make all fermented foods at home in this
essential book for your culinary library. Inside, you'll find recipes for making coleslaws,
preserved lemons, ceviche, vinegars, yogurt, and more. The science, art, and craft of
fermenting foods are also explained in meaningful detail"-- Provided by publisher.

ISBN 978-1-59253-784-6 (pbk.)
1. Fermented foods. 2. Fermentation. I. Title.
TP371.44.L485 2012
664'.024--dc23

2011050783

Design: Holtz Design
Layout: everlution design
Photography: Glenn Scott Photography
Cover Design: Holtz Design

Printed in China

To Mom and Dad,
who showed me how to eat and how to question.

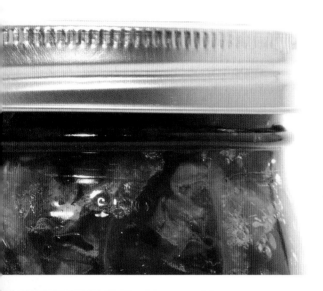

# CONTENTS

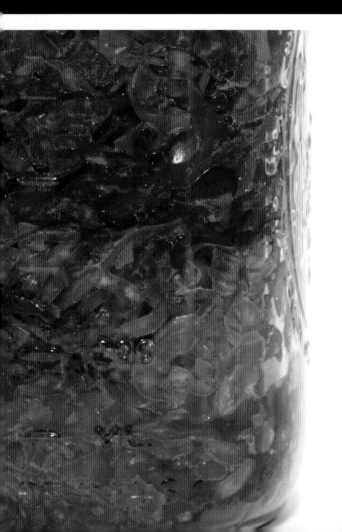

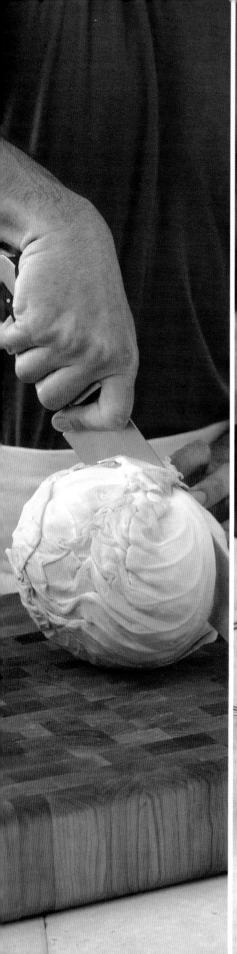
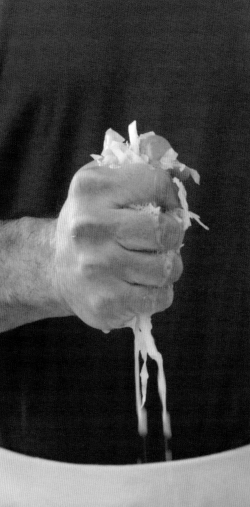
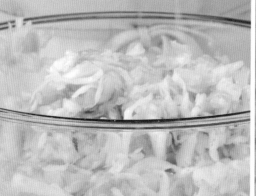
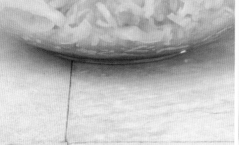
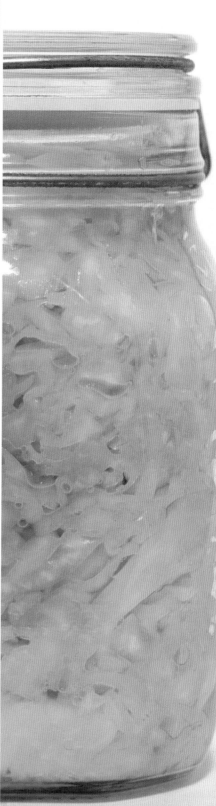

# INTRODUCTION: FERMENTATION JOURNEY

*I like changing things for the better.* I am curious about how things work. And I think a lot about food.

I love the idea of transforming food, in harmony with nature, as it has been done for thousands of years. Sauerkraut, for instance, need contain nothing more than cabbage and salt—no mysterious chemicals, no additives, not even any vinegar. So simple, yet so complex: Fermentation occurs because we seduce microscopic beings into doing our biochemical bidding, and they create sour acids that can preserve cabbage for many seasons.

I also love the process of making fermented foods. It is a checklist of gratifying activities. I go to a farmers' market or a farm, chat with food producers, and pay them a fair price for their work. I think creatively about what food I want to make. I craft the food myself, using whatever tools are available, sometimes improvising, and I often wind up with something great. In time, I get the reward of eating it—and sharing it with my community of friends and family.

When we make our own food, we regain some control over our lives—especially at a time in history when many of us feel at the mercy of events, governments, corporations, and industrial food producers. We also bridge the global gulf between the people who make food and the people who eat it, a gulf that perpetuates a grim litany of problems from famine and obesity to pollution, water shortages, wars over scarce resources, and deforestation.

I am delighted to share with you my passion for fermentation.

Take what you want from this book, experiment, and set out on your own food journey so that you might transform your food, your world, and yourself.

# HOW TO USE THIS BOOK

Each chapter has a specific focus. The first chapter is an overview of food preserving. Chapter 2 discusses choosing ingredients. Chapter 3 provides an in-depth look at making sauerkraut, and then chapter 4 broadens to other fermented vegetables. The remaining chapters walk you through fermenting dairy, fruit condiments, beverages, and meat.

Perhaps all you want to do is make fermented fruit chutney. With a typical cookbook, you might simply turn to the chutney recipe and follow it without reading the whole chapter. With this book, I encourage you to skim the entire chapter, or even the whole book, first! Knowledge is cumulative, and points made earlier in the book inform the recipes throughout.

People read books, especially cookbooks, in their own way. And many people don't want to be told how to read a book. But I do have reasons for making my suggestions.

If I've done my job right, then the early chapters will give you information to help you understand why the recipes work, some peace of mind about why they are safe, a better idea of what to do when things go wrong, and tools to help you decide how you might or might not want to modify the recipes as you continue to make them.

Recipes in some chapters depend on ingredients that you make in other chapters. When this is the case, I point it out, so of course you can jump back and forth and read the relevant sections as needed. Fermented fruit condiments, for instance, require a starter, and making sauerkraut and straining yogurt are two good ways to get a starter. If you've already read about making sauerkraut and straining yogurt, you will understand the starters you need for making fruit condiments. If you haven't, you might need to go back and read those sections again.

The more you have thought about the sources of your ingredients, the more satisfaction you may get out of a recipe, and in some cases, the better the recipe will work—and the healthier it will be. For this reason, you may find it useful to read the chapter about selecting ingredients, chapter 2, before you try any of the recipes. For instance, it is good to understand when chlorinated water can be a problem, along with ways that you can remove chlorine from water; when it's most important to avoid pesticide-treated fruit; and the relative merits of different kinds of salt.

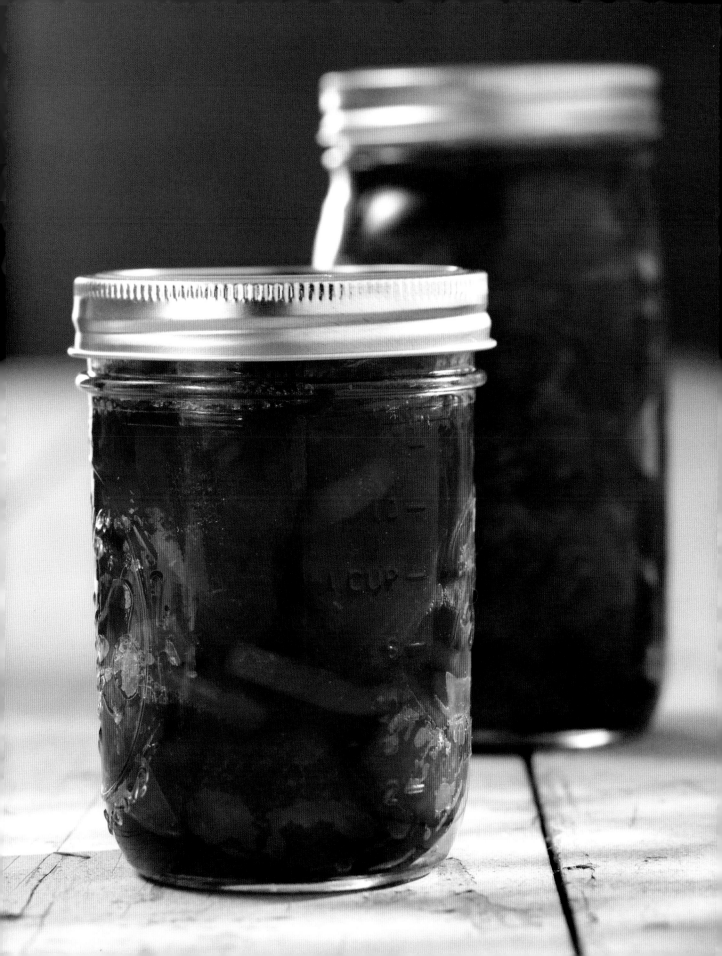

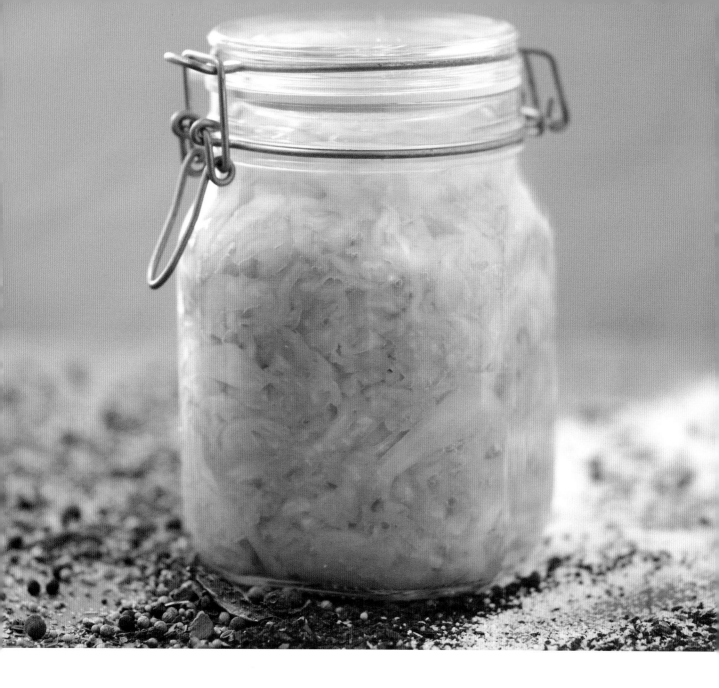

# PLAYING WITH OUR FOOD

The world around us is in upheaval. News media report wars, pandemics, famines, financial crises, tsunamis, meltdowns, and other calamities—natural and manmade. No sooner have we digested one than we must attempt to swallow the next.

Our individual lives are in turmoil as well. Personal time has become scarce, as never-ending parades of distractions compete for our attention. The Internet grants us unprecedented access to information, communication, entertainment, and ever more compelling ways to spend our time and money. This same Internet erodes our privacy and quietude.

Amidst all this, do we really have time to play with our food? Can we afford to spend hours in the kitchen and prepare our own food when there are "real problems" out there that we should perhaps be addressing? Or are we fermenting while Rome burns?

I believe that preparing food, with all that it entails—including thinking about it, playing with it, learning about it, preserving it, and particularly fermenting it—is an exceptionally worthy activity, not despite the problems in the world around us, but because of them.

So my answer is yes: we can—and should—play with our food.

## PRESERVING FOOD

Preserving food is an important aspect of food preparation. Food can be preserved in many ways. Some preserving methods are suitable for home, while others are feasible only in an industrial setting.

★ Drying and salting are two of the oldest preserving methods. All the method-specific ingredients are easy to get: salt, heat, and fresh air. Many types of food can be dried and/or salted, including fruits, grains, and fish and meats. In fact, humans have been growing grain for 10,000 years, and because growing grain does not make sense unless you dry it, we can conclude that humans have been drying food for at least 10,000 years.

★ Ultraviolet light, ionizing radiation, and high pressure are some of the newest tools for preserving food. Some food you buy in the store has been processed with these technologies: nuts and spices are often irradiated, for instance, and prepared foods like guacamole are sometimes treated with high pressure. These are not preserving techniques that you can employ at home.

★ Vinegar, acids like citric acid or ascorbic acid, and other preservative chemicals can be added to foods to help them remain edible longer. Home preservers use these additives, as do industrial food producers. Some preservative chemicals, such as sodium nitrite, may be bad for us, so I recommend avoiding them.

★ Canning is a food preserving technique that has been in use for approximately 200 years. It is a popular and practical way to preserve food, on both a small and a large scale. It is often used in conjunction with vinegar, acids, and other preservative chemicals.

★ Refrigeration is another popular food preserving technique. Before electricity was widely available, ice suppliers cut big blocks of ice from frozen lakes and shipped them to warmer areas, where they would be used to keep food cold. Things are easier today, at least in wealthy countries with electricity.

★ Freezing is one of the most popular long-term food preserving techniques today. It often requires a steady supply of electricity. It's only in the last hundred years that freezing food at home has become practical year-round. Many people freeze food every day without thinking of it as a preserving technique.

## FERMENTING: MY FAVORITE FOOD PRESERVING TECHNIQUE

Fermenting, last and definitely not least, is my favorite food preserving method. It is peculiarly well suited to the home food preserver and has been for a long time, in rich countries and in poor ones. Here's why:

**Fermenting is tolerant of imprecision.**
Fermentation can succeed even when there's variation in times, temperatures, and ingredient ratios. It is pretty difficult to get food poisoning from wrongly fermented foods.

Canning, by contrast, is much less tolerant of imprecision; it is a persnickety process, and failure to sterilize equipment properly, or to process canned food for the right length of time or at the right temperatures, can lead to serious food poisoning often with no telltale signs. This food poisoning is relatively rare these days because proper procedures are well documented and understood, but the specter of food poisoning makes me less inclined to improvise when canning—and that takes some of the fun out of it for me.

**Fermentation does not require expensive or unusual equipment, often requiring no special equipment whatsoever.** Many fermentation recipes rely only on vegetables, salt, a knife, and jars. Some recipes can be facilitated or expedited by the use of a food processor—making kimchi with only a knife, or with a mortar and pestle, can be time consuming, for instance—but power tools are never necessary. Fermentation can always be achieved without electricity, often without any source of energy at all besides arms and hands (and sometimes feet).

**Fermentation can be self-perpetuating.** By this I mean that when fermentation recipes do require special ingredients, they are often ingredients that can be created by fermenting other things. Because of this, fermentation is more sustainable, in the literal sense, than processes that require ingredients that might be hard to find, now or in the future, or that require industrial manufacturing. Many people made cider and wine before it was possible to buy packets of yeast in the store. Packets of yeast can save you time or trouble, but they are not necessary.

**Fermentation can enhance the nutritive value, healthfulness, and digestibility of foods.** The microbes responsible for fermentation often create enzymes and vitamins, break down difficult-to-digest food components, and make minerals more available for your body to assimilate. Fermentation is the best preserving method in this regard.

**Fermenting often improves the flavor of foods, although of course this is a matter of opinion!**
Not everyone would agree that blue cheese or ripe Camembert is an improvement over fresh milk, or that sauerkraut is an improvement over raw cabbage. Some fermented foods are acquired tastes; love can be a gradual thing.

Here is a loose, incomplete, and imperfect categorization of some fermented foods talked about in this book. For each category, I have chosen a representative, or an archetype, that embodies qualities of many of the other foods in that category. I hope this helps you navigate the territory of fermented foods and helps reveal the role that fermented foods play in our everyday lives. Without fermentation, most of our favorite foods and beverages would not exist!

## ARCHETYPES OF FERMENTATION

| CATEGORY | MICROBES | ARCHETYPE | OTHER EXAMPLES |
| --- | --- | --- | --- |
| Lacto-fermented vegetables and fruit | Bacteria | Sauerkraut | Pickles, kimchi, fermented vegetables, preserved lemons, salsas, chutneys |
| Fermented dairy | Bacteria (mostly), yeast, mold | Yogurt | Kefir, crème fraîche, sour cream, cultured butter, cheese |
| Alcoholic beverages | Yeast (mostly) | Cider | Mead, wine, beer, sake |
| Lacto-fermented beverages | Bacteria | "Ginger Ale" | Root beer, vegetable kvass, and other beverages fermented with whey and fermented vegetable juice as starters |
| Dual-fermented beverages | Bacteria, yeast | Vinegar | Kombucha, kefir, water kefir |
| Fermented meats | Bacteria (mostly), yeast, mold | Corned beef | Pickled meats, dry sausages, hams |
| Fermented fish | Bacteria | Fish sauce | Fermented shellfish, rakfish, surströmming |
| "Luxuries" | Bacteria (mostly) | Chocolate | Coffee, some kinds of tea |
| Fermented soy | Mold, bacteria, fungus | Soy sauce | Miso, tempeh, natto |
| Other | Bacteria | Olives | Capers and caperberries |

Beyond all of this, fermentation involves an element of magic, and an element of faith. In order to ferment our food, we conjure armies of invisible microbes to wage war against the forces of decay. We create the right conditions for them, by arranging for the right amount of salt, the right amount of air, the right temperature, and so on, and we must trust that the soldiers will arrive and ferment. Even in today's world of high-speed Internet and GPS navigation, I still get a little thrill each time my sauerkraut starts bubbling because I know that it means I have successfully seduced my microbes.

# CHAPTER 1
# FOOD PRESERVING (IN BRIEF)

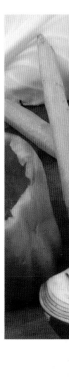

THIS CHAPTER DISCUSSES WHAT IT MEANS for food to spoil—both how we experience spoiled food and what processes cause it to spoil. Food preserving is everything that we do to prevent food from spoiling or to slow down the process. The conditions that cause food to spoil can be analyzed and broken down into various factors; I'll discuss each of these, as well as how you might seek to adjust them to prevent or postpone spoilage. Understanding all of these things will help you understand the mechanisms whereby various popular food preserving techniques, particularly fermentation, work.

It is worthwhile to look at food preserving in a somewhat technical and quantitative way; this helps us see why our preserved food is safe and how we can modify our recipes without compromising safety. For instance, if we know that acidity preserves food, we may feel comfortable replacing vinegar with lemon juice or kombucha in a recipe.

# WHAT IS FOOD PRESERVING?

Food preserving is *extending a food's window of edibility*. Edibility entails safety and palatability (including deliciousness).

Left to its own devices, food tends to spoil, more or less quickly depending on its type. A head of cabbage left out on the kitchen counter, for instance, might go some number of days before starting to dry out; insects might start to eat it, and, depending on the temperature and humidity, it might start to get moldy. In the summer, it certainly wouldn't be very appetizing after five or so days. By comparison, fermented cabbage can last weeks or months at room temperature—even longer if it is kept somewhere cool. Sailors used to take sauerkraut on long ocean voyages, and in Korea, kimchi is made in the fall and then eaten all winter and spring.

Fruit is even more perishable than cabbage: raspberries, for instance, can get moldy in less than a day, and peaches shrivel up even while getting mushy. Fresh grapes are best right after they've been picked and are pretty unappealing after sitting out for a week, but wine can have a shelf life of anywhere from one year to fifty years!

When trying to extend a food's window of edibility, you face challenges from a few sources:

**Other organisms that try to eat your food.**
Organisms, large and small, mammalian, single-celled, and everything in between, will try to eat your food. These organisms can range from rodents and insects to yeasts, molds, and bacteria. Depending on where you are, you may even be in competition with deer, coyotes, eagles, or bears. Some of these organisms are more visible than others. In fact, the microscopic ones live everywhere—in the air and the water and even on your skin; preventing them from eating your food can be difficult. Often the best you can hope for is to slow them all down, choose which ones of them will win, and to limit the success of the others.

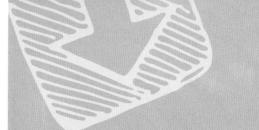

## WHY PRESERVE?

Why would we want to extend a food's window of edibility? There are many reasons why, historically, we have preserved food, and will continue to preserve it:

★ Hunter-gatherers of the past (as nearly all of them are) devoted relatively little time to food preserving; for the most part, they ate what was available, when it was available. If they could not find enough to eat in a given place, they moved somewhere else, or sometimes they suffered. If we preserve food, then we don't have to move when we run out of local, seasonal food.

★ The advent of agriculture, grains in particular, drew into sharp focus the problem of the uneven yield cycle: Much of the crop would be ready for harvest all at once, and there would be long gaps between harvests. This was particularly the case for people living in colder climates, where entire seasons go by with no new crops. Raising livestock for meat brought similar issues: It is better to have weeks or months to eat a cow, rather than being forced to eat it all at once. Thus, preserving allows food from a bounty to be consumed gradually.

★ When people started keeping animals for milk, the need arose for a way to preserve dairy products, since milk does not remain fresh very long in warm climates. This need led to the emergence of a broad range of dairy foods, including yogurt, kefir, butter, cheese, and so on. Most dairy foods can be looked at as "preserved milk" because they have a much longer room-temperature life expectancy than milk.

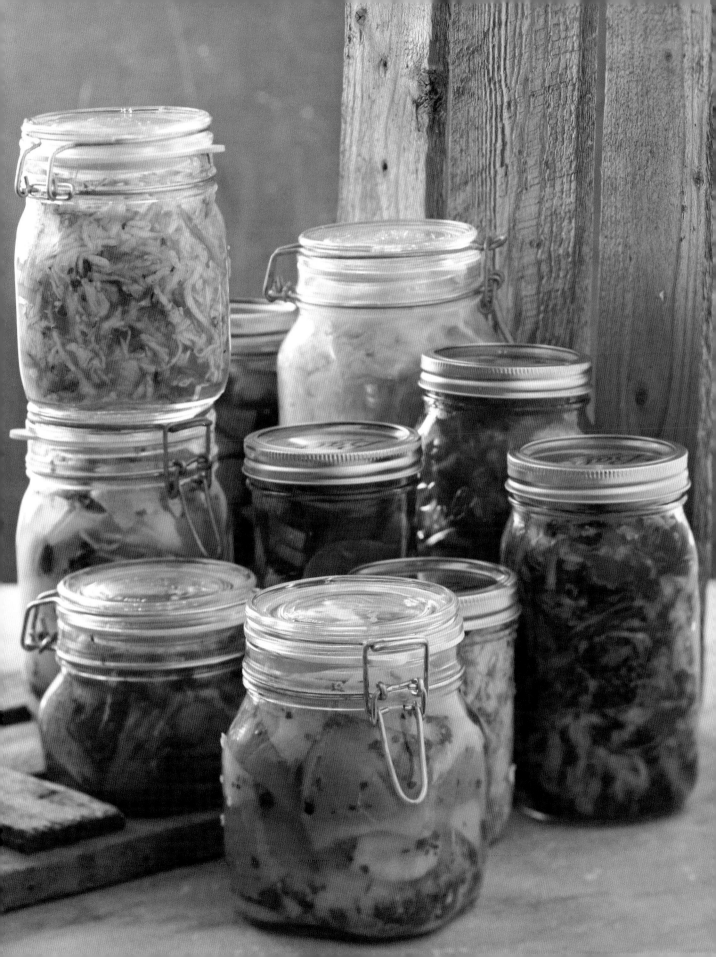

* Explorers, travelers, and specifically sailors have always had to carry supplies that would last for weeks or months. At some point, people figured out that they needed a variety of foods in order to avoid diseases of deficiency; for instance, sailors started bringing with them citrus juice, sauerkraut, and other foods containing vitamin C because vitamin C is protective against scurvy. Today's astronauts, whose diets are limited to what they take with them on their ships, have the same needs. Food preserving has allowed humans to travel places they could not otherwise have reached.

* As explorers traveled the world and societies mingled, demand arose for goods from faraway places, "exotic" goods that needed to be transported thousands of miles. (The word "exotic" derives from the Greek *exotikos*, meaning simply "from outside.") Tea and sugar cane are good examples; their monetary value and great popularity created a compelling incentive for their preservation and transportation.

* Even small amounts of alcohol are quite effective at killing potentially harmful microorganisms—and alcoholic beverages are products of fermentation. Thus, when safe drinking water has been scarce, as it was in parts of Europe during the Middle Ages, mild alcoholic beverages have been a useful option.

## ANCIENT MEANS, MODERN REASONS

Today, as always, transporting food over long distances necessitates preserving it. Folks in icy winters demand berries and lettuce, and landlocked eaters enjoy deep-sea fish almost as much as coast dwellers. What were once considered regional foods or luxury items are now widely available in all big cities and many towns. Refrigeration and freezing have fueled this trend, as have both traditional methods of preserving and newer preservation techniques that involve chemicals, pressure, and even radiation.

And while food preserving originated as a survival technique, and later became essential for travel and commerce, people gradually discovered and rediscovered that preserved food can be different from the original, and sometimes better.

New textures and flavors develop; wine, cheese, and bread are excellent examples. Digestive and nutritive benefits accrue; many preserved foods, such as fermented cassava (versus raw cassava), sauerkraut (versus raw cabbage), and natto (versus raw soybeans), are easier to digest and more nutritious than their fresh counterparts, sometimes dramatically so. In fact, raw soybeans and raw cassava can be toxic!

**Cellular breakdown.** In a living plant or animal, as quickly as old cells die off, break down, and are reabsorbed, new cells are created. The breakdown is mediated by enzymes, and the creation of new cells is made possible by the circulation throughout the body of energy and cellular building blocks. When an animal dies or a vegetable or fruit is picked, this circulation stops, so the existing cells continue to break down, but no new cells are created to replace them. The cellular breakdown manifests itself as the loss of water from cells and the weakening of cell walls. This is part of why old vegetables dry out or become mushy. Greens lose their crunchiness, tomatoes and other soft fruit get softer, and summer squash start to cave in.

**Oxidation.** Foods, especially those containing fats but also some others, are subject to oxidation when exposed to air. We see this when we cut a piece of raw meat or an avocado, an apple, or a potato, and it starts turning brown.

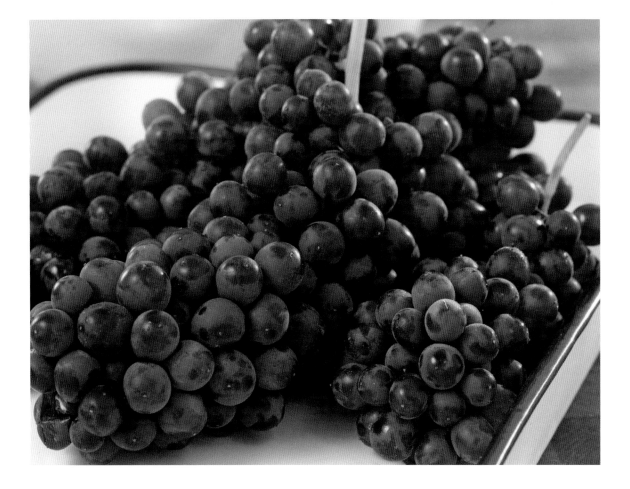

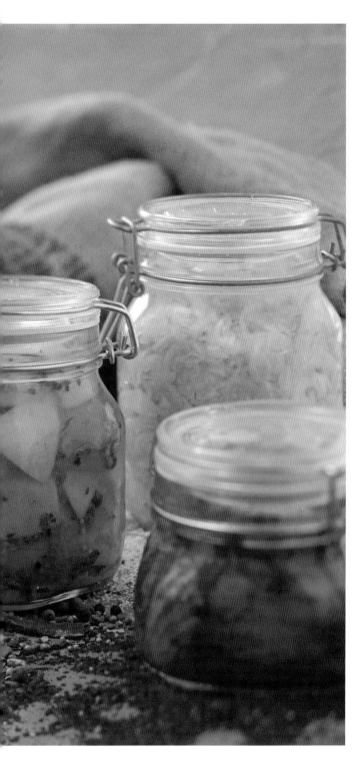

# THE ART AND CRAFT OF HOME PRESERVING

Preservers practicing their craft have brought us some of our most widely loved traditional foods. Almost every group of people around the world has its signature preserved foods, even if some of these foods aren't always recognized as preserved foods, and sometimes the modern versions of these foods differ from their originals. One people's favorite may seem intimidating or perhaps even horrifying to another people. Consider, in the chart on the next page, a small sample of the variety of fermented foods that the world's cultures contribute to our modern palates. Note that many of these foods are not limited to the regions mentioned.

Traditional fermented foods include coffee, some kinds of tea, chocolate, cheese, bread, wine, beer, cider, olives, pickles, chutney, sauerkraut, corned beef, sausage, natto, kimchi, sushi, ketchup, and many more.

## SOME SIGNATURE FERMENTED FOODS

| REGION/CULTURE | TRADEMARK FOOD | INGREDIENTS |
| --- | --- | --- |
| Central Europe | Sauerkraut | Cabbage, salt, and spices |
| Western, central, and southern Asia | Yogurt and kefir | Milk |
| Korea | Kimchi | Cabbage, salt, and spices |
| Southwestern Europe | Ham and dry sausage | Pork and salt |
| Europe | Wine | Grapes |
| Europe, Africa | Beer | Grain |
| Northern Europe and North America | Cider | Apples |
| Western Europe | Cheese | Milk and rennet |
| Japan | Miso | Soybeans |
| East Asia | Soy Sauce | Soybeans |
| North Africa, Southeast Asia | Preserved citrus | Citrus and salt |
| Southeast Asia, East Asia | Fish sauce | Fish and salt |
| Many places | Bread | Wheat and water |
| Southeast Asia, Africa, South America | Coffee | |

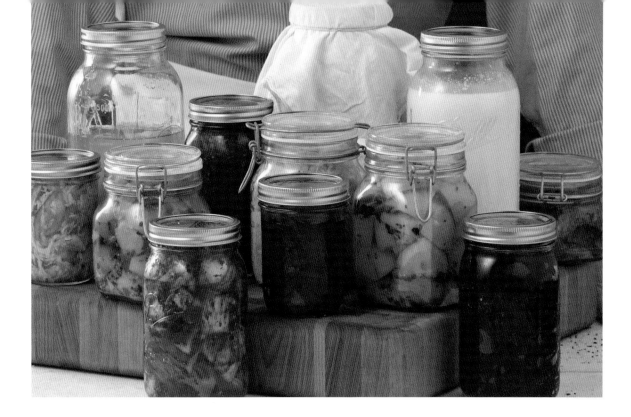

Motivations for preserving food at home extend beyond the general or historical inducements.

Making food "from scratch" allows you to choose raw materials produced by whatever methods you like, and gives you fine control over which techniques you apply and which additives you use. By contrast, commercial conglomerates choose raw materials, techniques, and additives based on profitability above all else. Their choices may be very different from what yours would have been and may not necessarily be disclosed.

Learning to preserve your own food also gives you valuable skills for a possible future in which the industrial food system may not be reliable. We don't know exactly what the future will bring, but we do know that populations are growing, water is getting scarce, fossil fuels are getting more expensive to extract, and our appetite for energy will only increase as more and more people in developing countries get cars. It is certain that the world will look different in fifty years, and it's quite conceivable that the global food economy will change radically.

Beyond these practical considerations, preserving food can be a creative activity, a craft that allows you to express yourself by making something unique. It's an endeavor that enables you to enjoy the satisfaction of making something by hand, bringing together a group of people around a common purpose and a shared meal, and reclaiming control over your own food destiny.

In past generations, food preserving was something that most people did. When a pig was slaughtered, the extended family, or even the entire village, came together to make sausages and hams. When tomatoes were picked, jars and jars of tomato sauce were made, to be consumed over the course of the next year. We can do the same thing today, whether we grow the ingredients ourselves, get them in season at the farmers' market, or just buy them at the store.

Bring your friends together, do some preserving, and trade some of your finished products.

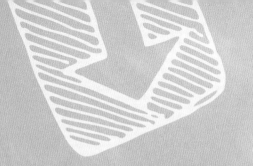

## THE THEORY OF PRESERVING FOOD

_____

Some microbes and enzymes cause food to decay, while others play a role in preserving it. In order to avoid decay, we must inhibit or destroy the decay-inducing agents. When you think about preserving, consider the following six factors that determine the ability of microbes, enzymes, and oxygen to act on food:

1. **The type of food.** In general, carbohydrates and proteins are hospitable to microbes; fats are not. This is why many oils and fats do not require refrigeration. (Fats can become rancid through exposure to heat, light, and oxygen, but this is not because of microbes; it is a purely chemical phenomenon.)

2. **Acidity.** Neutral and slightly acidic foods (a pH level between 4.6 and 7.5) are more hospitable to microbes; alkaline or strongly acidic foods are less so. Limes, for example, are very acidic (pH level 2) and so do not tend to spoil very quickly. Most vegetables are much less acidic (pH level between 5 and 7) and so, when left out, are more likely to decompose.

3. **Temperature.** Foods between the temperatures of 41°F (5°C) and 135°F (57°C) are more hospitable to bacteria than foods that are either very cold or very hot. Enzymes start getting deactivated and destroyed above 115°F (46°C).

4. **Time.** The longer a food is in the vulnerable zone of temperature or acidity, the more it will decay.

5. **Oxygen.** Environments that include air (oxygen, really) and airless environments welcome different kinds of microbes. Depending on your food preservation strategy, you might want to guarantee or constrain air supply. The bacteria that make vinegar, for example, need an environment that includes oxygen (aerobic) in order to go about their business; the bacteria that make sauerkraut prefer an environment that does not include oxygen (anaerobic).

6. **Moisture.** A water content between 85 and 97 percent is generally most hospitable to microbes. If we can make a food either too dry or too wet, we can keep decay at bay.

# WHY WE NEED MICROBES AND ENZYMES

Microbes are microscopic life forms, such as germs and fungi. Enzymes are proteins that catalyze and mediate various chemical processes that are necessary to keep organisms alive.

Some microbes are beneficial to humans, and some are harmful. Similarly, some enzymes are good for humans, and others are poisonous. Our bodies rely on bacteria, which are microbes, to help us digest food. In fact, a healthy human contains many more bacterial cells than human cells. When our bacterial colonies become depleted because of illness or antibiotic use, for instance, we need to rebuild these colonies. Eating live fermented foods is one way to do this; taking probiotic supplement pills is another.

Recently, the media have made people aware of the need for probiotics. Food manufacturers have seen an opportunity in this and have started highlighting their foods' probiotic attributes in their advertising. One manufacturer has gone so far as to develop its own specific strain of probiotic bacteria, patent this strain, add it to their yogurt, and then publicize its digestive benefits as if this were the first and only yogurt containing probiotic bacteria. They fail to mention that pretty much everyone else's yogurt contains probiotic bacteria, too. In fact, this manufacturer's yogurt contains sugars, fillers, and other unnecessary additives, so it is likely less beneficial to digestion than the humbler, less noisy yogurt next to it on the store shelf.

Some microbes are intrinsically antagonistic to humans and will cause our food to become unappetizing, or worse, toxic. When we eat toxic food and get sick, we call it food poisoning. Common sources of potentially deadly food poisoning are bacteria called *Salmonella, Clostridium botulinum*, which causes botulism, and *E. coli* O157:H7, which causes a potentially deadly type of colitis. (Notably, there are other strains of *E. coli* that occur naturally in our intestines and don't cause any problems at all.)

Our bodies rely on enzymes to help with vital processes such as digestion and metabolism. People who follow a "raw food" type of diet believe that we need all the enzymes we can get, and because heat destroys enzymes, they eat as much of their food as possible raw (or cooked at extremely low temperatures).

Enzymes, unchecked, will digest our food. Many of the same types of enzymes that occur in our mouths and in our digestive tracts also occur in the foods we eat. If we leave these foods out on the kitchen counter for too long, they will digest themselves. Amylases, for example, are enzymes that break down starches into sugars. These are what make fresh vegetables become less fresh, and these are what our bodies use to digest vegetables.

# WAYS TO DELAY DECAY

Different preserving methods use different strategies to fend off decay. These are some of the methods that can be used by the home preserver:

★ Refrigeration and freezing are effective because most microbes' metabolisms, and the actions of enzymes, slow greatly in the cold and essentially stop below freezing. Refrigeration and freezing do not gravely compromise the nutritional content of food, although the freeze/thaw cycle can burst food cell walls, affecting texture.

★ Packing in an acidic environment is a quick, cheap, and effective way of preserving food. This can be done via fermentation or by adding vinegar. Most microbes and enzymes cannot operate in a highly acidic environment. Other chemical preservatives such as sodium benzoate are sometimes used alongside acids. Some of these preservative chemicals can be harmful to us.

★ Packing in alcohol is another way to preserve food. A high-alcohol environment is effectively a low-moisture environment; microbes and enzymes are disabled or destroyed.

★ Drying, salting, and sugaring are ways of drawing water out of food, rendering it insufficiently moist for the activities of many kinds of microbes and enzymes.

★ Canning, whether in metal cans or in glass jars, relies on heat to destroy all microbes and enzymes, and relies on a hermetic seal to prevent microbes from reentering. The great virtue of canning is that when it is done properly, it can keep food for years. Its shortcomings are that (1) it can occasionally fail, and its failure can be disastrous, even fatal, because of the Clostridium botulinum (botulism) bacteria, and (2) the heat used in canning diminishes some heat-sensitive vitamins and destroys enzymes.

★ Meat that has been cooked to remove much of its moisture, salted to remove more, and then immersed in fat to create an anaerobic environment is called *confit*. It can keep for months.

★ Dairy has its own family of preservation techniques that variously convert sugars into acids, draw out water, isolate fat, and in some cases use heat to control bacteria and enzymes.

★ Fermentation underlies many of the techniques already listed. Vinegar and alcohol are both products of fermentation, and most ways of preserving dairy involve fermentation.

## NEW FRONTIERS IN FOOD PRESERVATION

New technologies, such as ultraviolet irradiation, high-pressure processing, and pulsed electric field processing, are now being used to sterilize food. Some of these technologies have been unleashed on the public after minimal testing and with little fanfare. Ideally, we could wait twenty years or so, see what unforeseen consequences emerge, weigh the costs and benefits, and then decide for ourselves which of these methods seem safe. Unfortunately, full disclosure is the exception rather than the rule, and unless we are acquiring food directly from its producer, it can be hard to tell how it may have been processed.

## CASE STUDY: APPLES

- - - - - - - - - - - - - - - - - - - - - - - - - - - - - -

What are the possible fates of an apple?

If you let an apple drop from its tree, it will likely get eaten by worms, birds, small land animals, or large land animals (like bears!). Or, especially if it is damaged in its fall from the tree branch, it might succumb to bacteria, yeasts, and molds. The exposed flesh is also likely to oxidize (turn brown), and, depending on the weather conditions, the apple might start to shrivel and dry up.

If you like, you can create a brighter future for this apple.

First, you can pick it carefully and store it somewhere moist and cool or cold (but not freezing). Under the right conditions, fresh apples can be stored for months.

Alternatively, you can core and slice the apple, and then put it in a hot, dry place until it is dehydrated. You can dry it until its texture is like that of leather, or until it is like that of a potato chip, or somewhere in between. If you do this and keep it somewhere dry, it can last for months.

You can purée the apple, perhaps add some lemon juice, heat it, put it in a jar, heat it some more, and then put it on a shelf. By doing this, you will have canned it. It will keep for a very long time, but you will have lost more of its natural vitamins and enzymes than in any of these other scenarios.

Finally, you can ferment the apple. Depending on what you're interested in doing, you might mix the apple with other fruit or vegetables and spices, introduce the right kinds of bacteria, and thus produce a chutney. Or you might juice the apple, introduce some yeast (or cross your fingers), wait a week or two, and produce some nice hard apple cider.

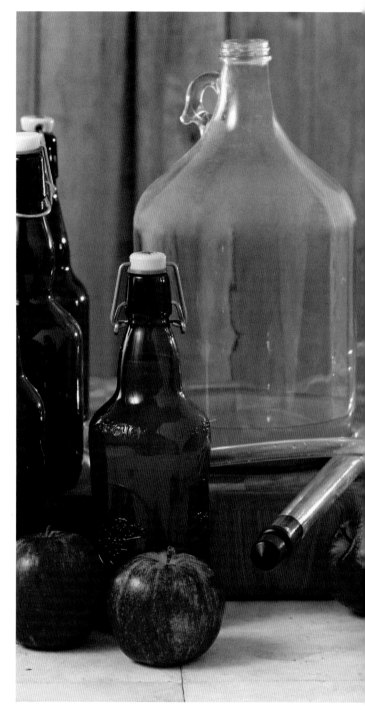

CIDER-MAKING EQUIPMENT

## CASE STUDY: CABBAGE

Consider the many different possible fates of a picked cabbage. The first, and least appetizing, option is to pick it and leave it out in the field on a warm day. There it may be partly eaten by animals or insects. It may also start to decompose, or rot, which is to say it may be partly eaten by microbes of various sorts or dissolved by its own enzymes.

As a home cook, you have these other options for processing the cabbage:

**It can be cooled:** If it is kept somewhere isolated at a low temperature, like in a refrigerator or a cellar, its rate of decay will be slowed greatly.

**It can be canned:** If it is heated and sealed under pressure in a sterile airtight container, it will reach a stable state that it might maintain for months or years.

**It can be fermented:** But if it is packed in salty liquid, and if other conditions are right, then it will follow a course that is a sort of middle road between rotting and canning—perhaps the best of both worlds. It will be eminently edible, and at the same time it will be a fertile playground for benign microbes. We call this fermentation.

## CASE STUDY: MILK

Most of us have been told not to leave milk out on the counter because it will spoil. This is a bit of an oversimplification of what happens, but regardless, there are other things you can do with milk besides keeping it out on the counter or putting it in the refrigerator.

If you skim the cream off the top of whole milk (assuming the milk has not been homogenized) and use just the cream, you can make butter, which will keep longer than milk.

If you introduce particular colonies of bacteria and then keep everything warm, you can make a durable, digestible, probiotic-rich, sour dairy food called yogurt.

By adding other things, heating it, separating the milk in various ways, and perhaps aging the result, you can produce a wide variety of other fermented dairy products, including cheeses.

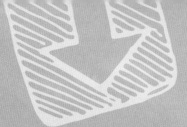

## BACTERIA VERSUS YEAST VERSUS BOTH

The term "microbe" can refer to any microscopic organism. The microbes responsible for most of our favorite fermented foods are bacteria and yeast. A few fermented foods (sake, some cheeses, some meat products, and some soy products) also rely on specific molds and other fungi to achieve their unique end points. Note that yeasts and molds are both types of fungi, along with mushrooms.

In general, yeasts consume sugars and produce alcohol, while bacteria consume sugars, starches, or alcohol and produce acids. Both alcohol and acids play roles in food preserving.

As foods become acidic, they become inhospitable to most kinds of microbes. Fortunately for us, the microbes that can survive in acidic environments are safe for us to eat: many of them are microbes that live within our bodies, and many of them are bacteria that enhance our digestion.

Food that contains more alcohol contains less water, which can make it less hospitable for some kinds of microbes. Also, alcohol itself is toxic to some microbes. In high enough concentrations, alcohol is toxic even to alcohol-producing yeasts, so 20 percent, or thereabouts, is the upper limit on alcohol content for a fermented beverage. To get a higher alcohol content than that, it's necessary to use the process of distillation, which separates the alcohol from the water by taking advantage of alcohol's lower boiling point. This is how stronger alcoholic beverages like brandy and vodka are made.

## FAVORITE FERMENTED FOODS AND THEIR FAVORITE MICROBES

| BACTERIA | YEAST | MOLD |
| --- | --- | --- |
| Sauerkraut | Sake | Sake |
| Kimchi | Wine | Cheese (some) |
| Pickles | Beer | Soy sauce |
| Other fermented vegetables | Cider | Tempeh |
| Yogurt | Mead | |
| Cheese (some) | Bread | |
| Kefir | Kefir | |
| Vinegar | Vinegar | |
| Kombucha | Kombucha | |

# WHEN IS A FOOD *PRESERVED*?

Fermentation is the metabolic transformation of foods via the action of microbes. These microbes are generally bacteria and yeasts, and they act primarily on the carbohydrate (sugar) content of foods.

When is a food *preserved*? We can consider fermented food to be preserved once it has reached a state where "unfriendly" microbes are kept in check by both the chemistry of the environment and the robustness of the friendly microbes, and enzymatic breakdown is inhibited.

If we are crafty, we can create conditions under which food will ferment in such a way as to preserve *itself*, with a minimum of human interference. We don't necessarily have to add acids or alcohol to the food ourselves; we can enlist and encourage the microbes to do this for us. And if all goes well, the resultant food will be at least as tasty as it was before it underwent its transformation.

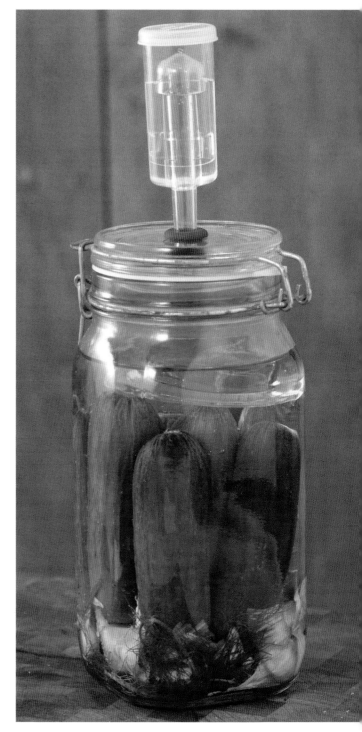

CUCUMBER PICKLES (RECIPE ON PAGE 82)

# AN OVERVIEW OF FERMENTATION: GETTING TO KNOW THE PROCESS

How exactly do you ferment food?

→ First, you need the food medium itself, which must contain some carbohydrates. This food may be vegetables or vegetable juice, fruits or fruit juice, grains, dairy, or even meat. You can also add carbohydrates to foods (often in the form of sugar), and then ferment the result; kombucha, for instance, is made from sugar-sweetened tea.

→ Next, you need the microbes, which you may get from any number of sources:

  1 the surface of the food, as part of the normal course of the food's life (especially in the case of fresh cabbage and its relatives like turnips and other *Brassica* vegetables)

  2 material from a previous round of fermentation, either similar or not to the fermentation you're attempting (for example, using yogurt to start yogurt, sauerkraut juice to start sauerkraut, or the liquid whey that separates from yogurt to start a fruit chutney)

  3 an envelope of microbes sold just for this purpose

→ Next, in some cases, you may choose to stack the deck further in favor of the desired microbes by adding salt. Salt pulls moisture out of foods, creates liquid, and inhibits many undesirable microbes.

→ You should consider whether or not you want the fermenting foods to be exposed to air, and package them accordingly. Sauerkraut, for example, should be protected from the air, especially early on in its fermentation, while kombucha and vinegar need air in order to brew.

→ You'll need a (relatively) dark place with an appropriate temperature so that your fermentation can thrive. Sunlight is generally bad for the bacteria and yeast that you'll be courting. Ideal fermentation temperatures vary from 50°F (10°C) to 110°F (43°C), depending on the food and the particular microbes involved. Some popular cool places for storing fermented foods include cellars (for pickles), caves (for cheese), and holes in the ground (for kimchi).

→ Finally, you need time, so that our little friends can work their magic. The amount of time varies from a couple of days to a couple of months or even longer.

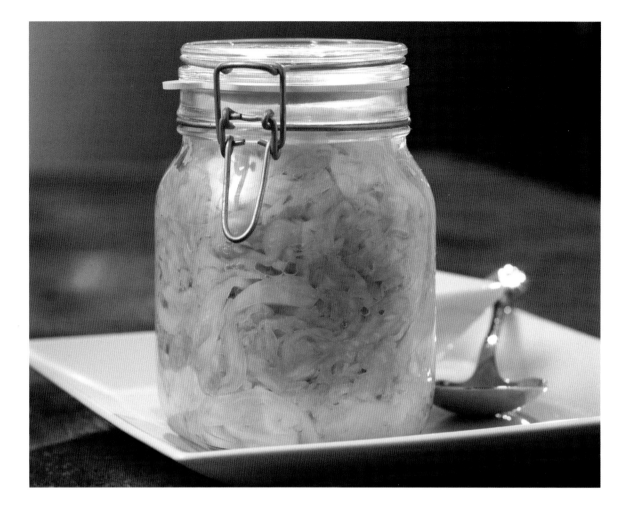

## FERMENTATION TIME AND TEMPERATURE

| FOODSTUFF | FERMENTATION TIME | FERMENTATION TEMPERATURE |
| --- | --- | --- |
| Sauerkraut and Kimchi | 4 days–4 months | 50°F (10°C)–80°F (30°C) |
| Yogurt | 12–24 hours | 100°F (40°C)–115°F (45°C) |
| Kefir | 12–24 hours | 50°F (10°C)–100°F (40°C) |
| Cheese | days–months | varies |
| Hard Apple Cider | 1–6 weeks | 40°F (5°C)–70°F (20°) |
| Kombucha | 5–15 days | 70°F (20°C)–85°F (30°C) |

 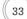

# HEALTH BENEFITS OF FERMENTATION

Some methods of food preserving affect the nutritional profile of foods negatively. Canning, for instance, relies on heating foods to the point where all microbes are destroyed; unfortunately, heat destroys the enzymes in food that help us digest them, and diminishes or destroys many vitamins (probably vitamins A, C, D, E, and some B vitamins, although there is some disagreement). Most other forms of preserving have some negative impact on nutrient content.

Many preservative chemicals have negative impacts on health; some of them are known carcinogens. Nonetheless, these chemicals remain in our food supply, and large-scale food processors use them because they are cheap and because they remove uncertainty from the food manufacturing process, usually by killing microbes or inhibiting enzymes.

And new techniques like irradiation, high-pressure processing, and pulsed electric field processing are not well understood; many people see serious problems with them or anticipate that we will discover serious problems with them.

By contrast, fermentation actually enhances food's nutritional value because it:

**Preserves nutrients.** Fermentation, because it does not involve high heat, preserves the vitamins and enzymes present in foods. In fact, beyond simply maintaining the vitamin content of raw foods, the process of fermentation can actually create new vitamins, specifically B vitamins and vitamin $K_2$, as well as some types of enzymes.

**Provides beneficial bacteria = a happy body.** The friendly microbes that carry out the fermentation process are often themselves beneficial to humans. Plain, whole-fat yogurt, for instance, is an excellent probiotic supplement that is available in most supermarkets (the more processed kinds of yogurt aren't as healthy). Recent research is confirming what alternative practitioners have been saying for some time: Friendly bacteria in the digestive tract are crucial to a properly functioning immune system.

**Helps the body digest carbohydrates.** Fermentation breaks down certain types of carbohydrates that can be difficult to digest. Raw cabbage, for instance, contains polysaccharides that can lead to intestinal gas; these polysaccharides are generally broken down by fermentation, leading to a less dramatic eating experience. Likewise, some people cannot drink pasteurized milk because their bodies lack the enzymes necessary to digest lactose (milk sugar); many of these same people have no problems with yogurt, hard cheeses, or sour cream, all of which contain significantly less lactose. (Many of these people may also be able to easily digest unpasteurized milk because it contains lactase, the enzyme required to digest lactose. This enzyme is destroyed when milk is pasteurized.)

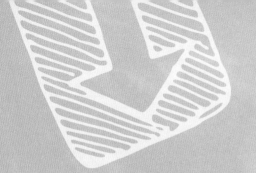

## KEY BENEFITS OF FERMENTING FOOD

Fermented food:

* preserves, sometimes even enhances, vitamin content of food

* preserves, sometimes even enhances, enzyme content of food

* is a healthy alternative to preservative chemical additives, some of which are toxic

* is a healthy alternative to high-tech preserving technologies, many of which are untested

* makes nutrients in foods more available to the body

* makes food less likely to cause digestive problems

## "FERMENTED" VERSUS "PICKLED"

Not all pickles are fermented, and not all fermented foods are pickled. But there is a lot of overlap.

In practice, "pickled" foods are foods that have been preserved in an acid medium. Fresh vegetables can be submerged in an acidic liquid like vinegar, resulting in vegetables that are pickled, but not fermented (although vinegar itself is created via a fermentation process, so vinegar pickles actually do rely, indirectly, on fermentation).

Fermented vegetables generally create their own acidic liquid as a result of the fermentation, so it is safe to say that fermented vegetables are both fermented and pickled.

Finally, there are alcoholic fermented foods like wine and apple cider that are fermented but not pickled. (Although when a person is drunk, we may speak of him or her as being "pickled," so nothing is cut and dried except of course foods that *have been* cut and dried.)

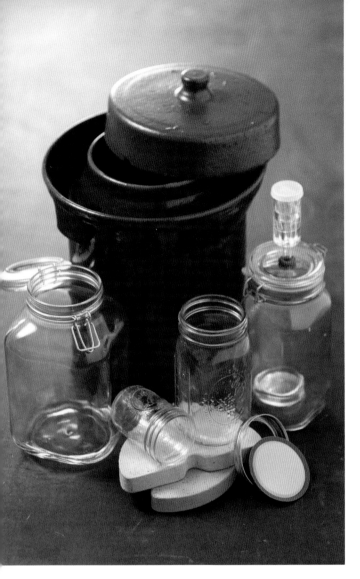

A VARIETY OF CONTAINERS FOR FERMENTING. *CLOCKWISE FROM TOP LEFT*: A SWING-TOP JAR; AN EARTHENWEAR HARSCH CROCK; A PICKL-IT FERMENTING JAR, WITH AIRLOCK; A COUPLE OF BALL JARS; WEIGHTS FOR THE HARSCH CROCK.

# STOCKING YOUR SCIENCE LAB

In my experience, Ball jars are suitable for fermenting cut and shredded vegetables, chutneys, salsas, yogurt, and most other things. The Pickl-It is great for all of these, as well as for whole vegetables, cucumber pickles, and items that are trickier and/or need to be weighted in order to be held below the surface of the liquid. I have not found the Harsch crock to be uniquely helpful for any particular project, and because it is bulky and expensive, it may not be the right tool for some people.

Big strainers and colanders are much more convenient than smaller ones when washing or rinsing large vegetables. Stainless steel surfaces are better than aluminum for kitchen tools for a variety of reasons: unlike aluminum, stainless steel is nonreactive, nontoxic, and dishwasher safe.

Buy the largest chef's knife that you can comfortably wield: 8 inches (20 cm) and 10 inches (25 cm) are both good sizes. If you are cutting a big vegetable, you are much better off with a big knife, and big knives can chop more food per stroke than smaller knives can.

The Star peeler is my favorite vegetable peeler.

Rounded saucepans make stirring and cleaning easier than pans, with creases; pots and pans made with aluminum cores heat more uniformly than do solid stainless pans and heat up and down the sides rather than just on the bottom. (It is best to avoid having aluminum touching your food for long periods of time, especially if your food is acidic.) The Calphalon Tri-Ply (pictured at right) is a great medium-size saucepan.

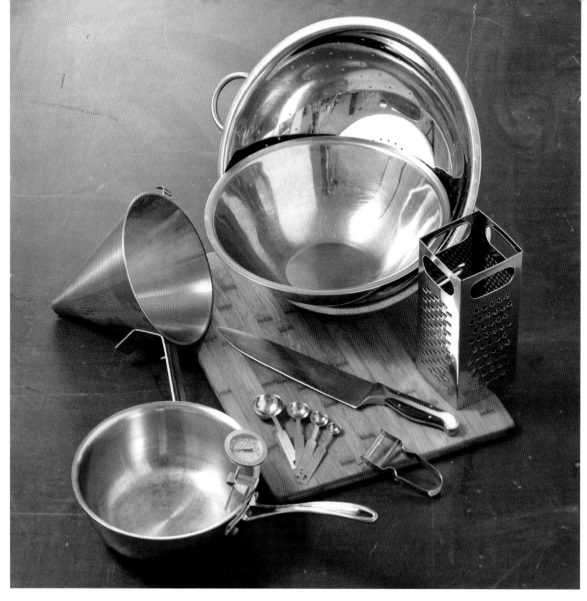

USEFUL KITCHEN TOOLS. *CLOCKWISE FROM TOP LEFT:* A CONICAL STRAINER; A MIXING BOWL; A LARGE COLANDER; A BOX GRATER; A 10-INCH (25-CM) CHEF'S KNIFE; A STAR VEGETABLE PEELER; MEASURING SPOONS; A STAINLESS STEEL INTERIOR, MULTI-PLY, ALUMINUM CORE, ROUNDED SAUCEPAN; A CHEESE-MAKING THERMOMETER; A WOODEN CUTTING BOARD.

The thermometer pictured above comes with a clip that allows you to attach it to the side of your pan in such a way that the tip of the thermometer is suspended in the liquid and does not touch the bottom or the sides of the saucepan. Thus, you can measure the temperature of the liquid rather than the temperature of the pan (which is likely to be hotter).

Wood is the best material for cutting boards because it is nontoxic; it does not dull your knives; and, according to some research, it is easier to clean and less likely than plastic to host malevolent microbes. (Also, it is pretty.) Do not cut directly on stainless steel, glass, or stone surfaces because these will dull your knives.

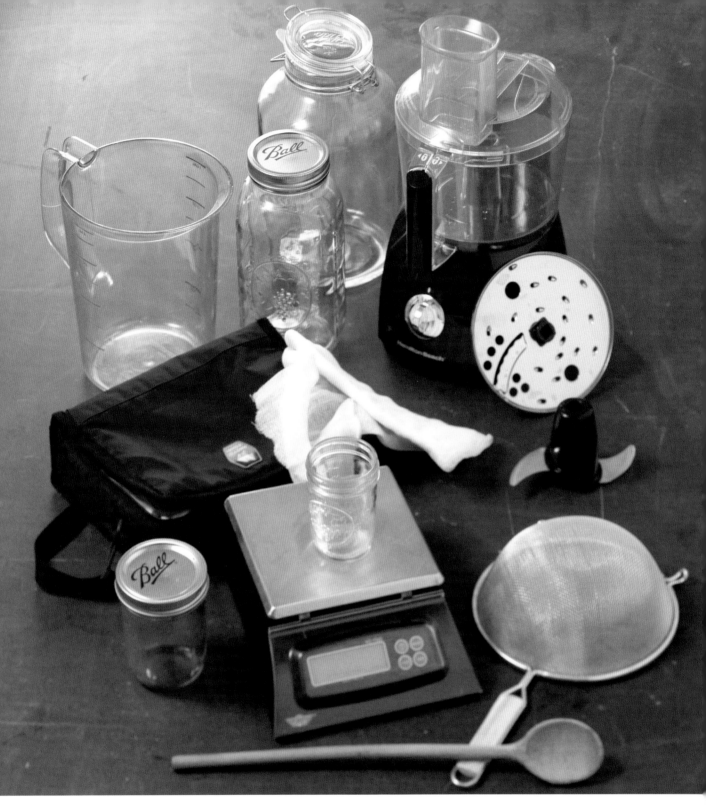

MORE FERMENTATION EQUIPMENT. *CLOCKWISE FROM TOP LEFT:* AN INSULATED
LUNCH BAG (USEFUL FOR MAKING YOGURT); A GALLON (4L) PITCHER; VARIOUS BALL
AND SWING-TOP JARS; A FOOD PROCESSOR, WITH SLICER WHEEL; A STRAINER; A
WOODEN SPOON; A DIGITAL FOOD SCALE; SOME CHEESECLOTH.

If you find yourself chopping or shredding a lot of food on a regular basis, consider investing in a food processor. It will save you a lot of time—and perhaps a shredded finger or two. If you enjoy fermenting or baking, or if you frequently find yourself cooking from recipes, a modern digital food scale is wonderful because it allows you to weigh your ingredients with great accuracy.

A 10-quart (9.4-L) stainless steel (not aluminum) stockpot is the smallest stockpot you should consider and may even be too small for some activities, like heating a large batch of milk for making cheese; heating a large batch of liquid in the process of brewing cider or beer; or making a large batch of stock from chicken or beef bones. You can buy carboys at specialized home-brewing stores, in person, or over the Internet; the one pictured here was originally a glass gallon cider bottle that I bought at the supermarket. An auto-siphon is another item that you are most likely to find at a home-brewing store; it allows you to pump liquid out of a large bottle without disturbing the sediment at the bottom.

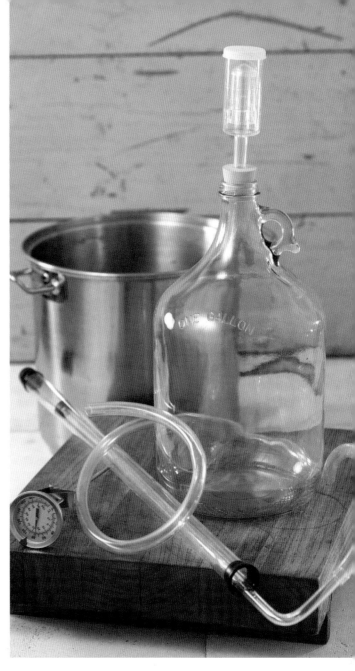

SOME CHEESE-MAKING AND BREWING EQUIPMENT. *CLOCKWISE FROM TOP LEFT:* A 10-QUART (9.4-L) STAINLESS STEEL STOCKPOT; A 1-GALLON (3.8-L) CARBOY WITH AIRLOCK; AN AUTO-SIPHON; A THERMOMETER; A WOODEN CUTTING BOARD.

# CHAPTER 2

# KNOW YOUR INGREDIENTS

CHOOSING THE BEST INGREDIENTS is key to having your creations turn out as delicious and nutritious as possible.

Many factors help determine what the "best" ingredients are. Freshness is one: Generally, the fresher your ingredients, the better the result. This often means choosing food produced locally and in season. Production method is another: Food produced with a minimum of industrial inputs will taste better and be better for you. Organic can be helpful, but it is not the whole story. The genetics of the food itself are important: Genetically modified foods are recent creations, and there are already signs that they are not at all the same as their traditional counterparts. Insufficient testing was done before they were unleashed on the public, so unless you would like to be part of the ongoing test, they are best avoided.

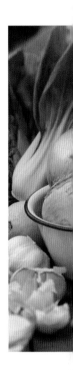

For nonanimal, nonvegetable ingredients, chemical purity is a factor. If a recipe calls for water, then the purer the water, the better. Chlorine, for instance, is found in much of the municipal water supply and should be removed, both because it is bad for you and because it can get in the way of fermentation. Likewise, much of the salt sold at the supermarket contains chemicals that are added to prevent it from clumping, or for other reasons; unfortunately, these chemicals can taste bad, be unhealthy, or, worst of all, impede your fermentation!

The best way to be certain about the provenance, paternity, and purity of your ingredients is to make your food from scratch when possible. This is one of the greatest things you can do for yourself, for your community, and for your family.

# THE FRESHNESS FACTOR

Fresher ingredients are generally better. Here's why.

★ Raw food naturally contains enzymes. From the moment vegetables are picked, these enzymes start to break them down and make them mushy. (The same thing happens with meat, although some amount of breakdown can actually improve the texture of meat.)

★ Certain flavors and vitamins in food decay over time when exposed to heat, light, and air.

★ As food sits around, microbes and other things start nibbling on it. If we don't take precautions, bacteria, molds, fungi, yeasts, insects, rodents, bears, and so on can eat our food, or render it unsafe for human consumption.

FRESH, ORGANIC NAPA CABBAGE,
FIT TO BE FERMENTED.

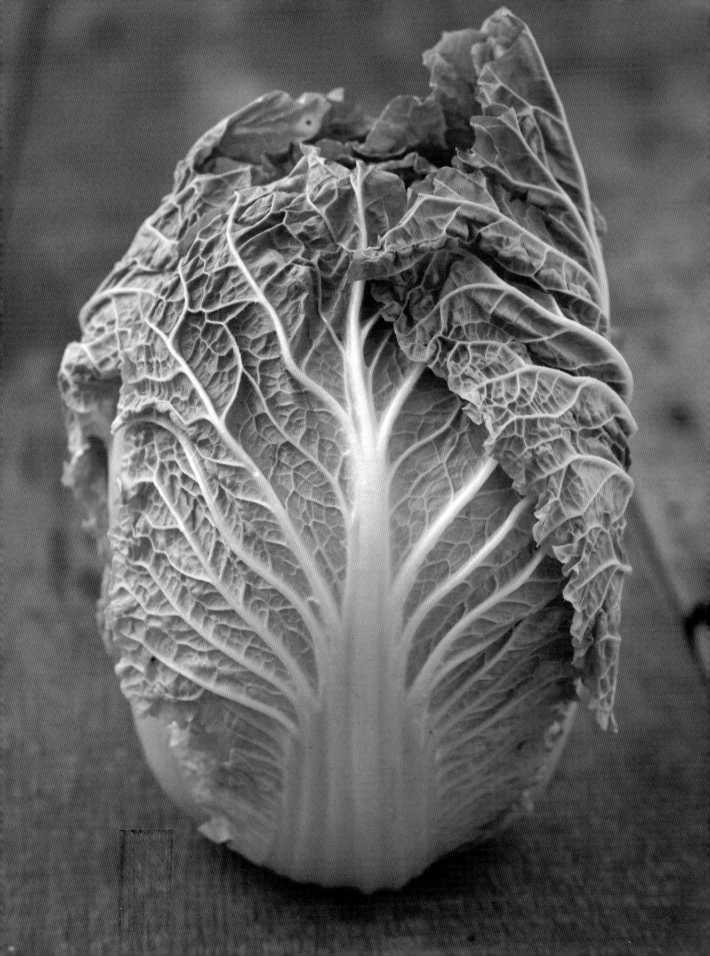

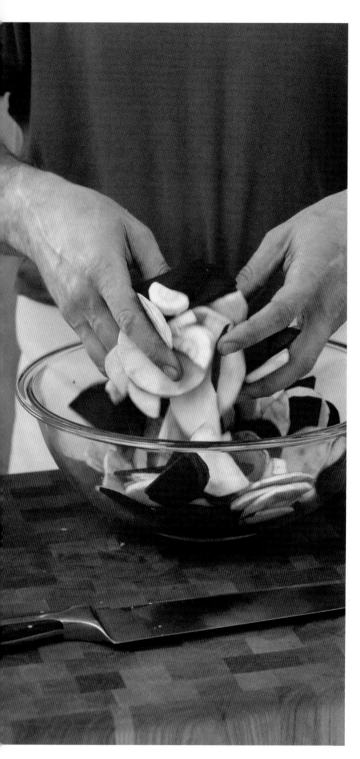

## BUYING LOCAL AND IN SEASON

When you buy vegetables at a farmers' market, you can ask the vendor when the vegetables were picked, where they were grown, what farming methods were used, and so on.

When you buy vegetables at a supermarket, you may not be able to get this information—and the vegetables will probably have been sitting around longer, especially if they came from far away. You can usually find out what country the vegetables are from, but often not much more.

## BUYING ORGANIC

In the United States, products labeled "Organic," "USDA Organic," or "100% Organic" are legally required to have been produced in particular ways. Only specific types of fertilizers, pesticides, and herbicides can be used, and producers must pay fees to qualified certification agencies.

Outside the United States, countries, unions, and jurisdictions have similar labeling laws. For instance, any products marked with the EU organic logo are subject to certain requirements regarding inputs, inspections, and certifications.

Before "organic" acquired legal meanings, it was used colloquially to describe food produced in a "natural" way, without industrially produced treatments or soil amendments.

SLICED RED BEETS AND TURNIPS ARE
COMBINED FOR A LATE-SPRING BATCH
OF BRINED VEGETABLES.

The problem with the old, informal system was that it was not specific, was not regulated, and was a matter of trust. The problem with the new, official system is that small producers may not be able to pay the certification fees without financial hardship. Also, the new system creates a simple dichotomy—organic versus nonorganic—that can mask some of the food's other characteristics that may also be important, such as locality, seasonality, and time to market.

Having said all of this, it is still true that in a supermarket, organic is usually better than nonorganic.

Buying organic vegetables and fruit is particularly important when:

1   you plan to eat the rind, peel, skin, or outermost portions of the food (as you might with apples, grapes, soft fruit, or citrus);

2   you are buying particular types of food that either tend to get a lot of pesticides applied to them or tend to absorb pesticides (such as bell peppers, celery, collard greens, and apples);

3   some of your eaters are sick, old, or have weakened or sensitive immune systems.

The Environmental Working Group publishes a "Shopper's Guide to Pesticides in Produce," which can be helpful in assessing some of the potential risks of non-organic fruit and vegetables.

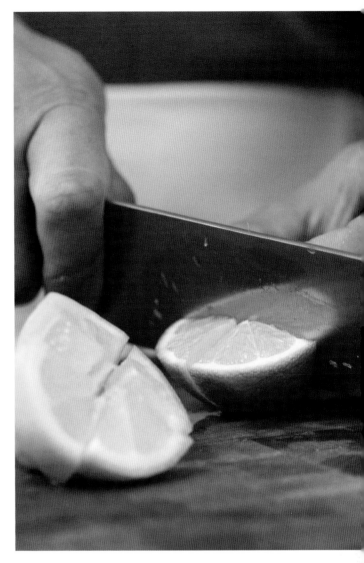

CITRUS FRUIT IS A VERY REGION-SPECIFIC CROP, AND CLOSE CONVERSATIONS WITH THE GROWER BEFORE BUYING MAY NOT BE AN OPTION.

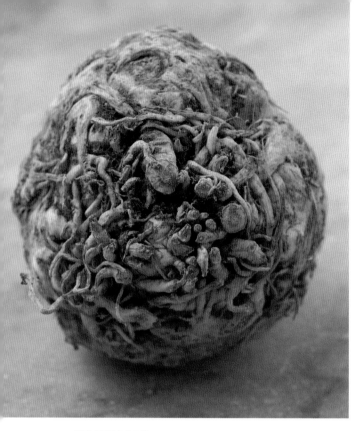

CELERY ROOT

When you are able to talk to a food producer—at a farmers' market, for instance—you can have a longer conversation about farming practices, why something may or may not be certified organic, why the producer made specific decisions, and so on. "Certified organic" does not always mean "more natural," particularly in the case of meat, eggs, and dairy. For example, certified organic eggs can be laid by chickens who practically never go outside and never eat the bugs and worms that they need for optimal health, while small, local farms may produce eggs that are more nutritious, fresher, and better in almost every way, but are not certified organic.

Similarly, organic vegetables produced and processed on a large scale can have more opportunity to become contaminated during picking, processing, packing, and shipping than vegetables from a small local farm.

## GENETICALLY MODIFIED

Genetically modified organisms (GMOs) are those whose DNA has been modified in a laboratory. DNA is the blueprint for all living things. By splicing in pieces of DNA from different species, often very different ones, scientists aim to engineer the characteristics of a particular genetically modified plant or animal. For instance, a significant fraction of corn sold in the United States today contains DNA from a species of bacteria named *Bacillus thuringiensis*; this alteration makes the corn toxic to certain pests. The supposed advantage of the modification is that it decreases the "need" for spraying pesticides on this crop.

Some scientists, including of course those working for the companies that develop and sell GMO technology, claim that eating genetically modified (GM) food is safe. Other scientists believe that GM food is dangerous and has contributed to a variety of singularly modern problems, including allergies, autoimmune diseases, decline of bee populations, and so on. They also point out that the GM food regulatory approval process is far too short and maintain that because of this, we can't properly assess the long-term effects of GM foods on human, animal, or plant populations, or on the ecosystem as a whole.

It may be prudent to avoid genetically modified foods until we see which side wins this debate. At the very least, you might consider evaluating the competing arguments yourself before making a decision about whether or not you want to eat GM foods—or really, continue eating them, because if you haven't been paying *very* close attention, you've been eating them for years.

If you decide to avoid GM foods, the next step is to identify which foods have been genetically modified.

★ In many countries, including most of Europe and Russia, GM foods are required to be labeled as such.

★ The United States has no requirement for specific labeling of GM foods, but basic food items that are certified organic are guaranteed not to be genetically modified. Processed foods labeled "100% organic" are guaranteed not to contain GM ingredients—but if they are merely labeled "organic," they *may* contain some percentage of ingredients derived from GM foods.

★ The variety of GM foods approved for human consumption changes from year to year, as do surrounding regulations.

Up-to-date information about GM foods, including arguments for and against, can be found in scientific journal articles. But the most significant new findings get summarized and discussed on the Internet immediately; that's where the public dialogue occurs, and it's probably the best place to find the latest news.

## WATER

Some fermentation recipes call for the use of water or brine. Municipal tap water can contain varying amounts of chlorine and/or a related chemical called chloramine. These are added by the water authorities to prevent the propagation of microbes of various sorts. Chlorine and chloramine do this very well. The problem is that successful fermentation depends on the propagation of microbes! So for fermenting purposes, it is good to remove as much chlorine and chloramine as possible from the water.

There are various ways to try to remove chlorine and chloramine from water. These work to varying degrees.

★ Leave the water out in an open container for 12 to 24 hours. This allows chlorine to come out of solution with the water and escape into the air. It works less well with chloramine.

★ Boil the water for a couple of minutes and allow it to cool. This forces chlorine gas to boil away.

★ Use a carbon water filter (pitcher filter, faucet filter, or under-sink filter).

★ Use a reverse osmosis filter. These are available at most home improvement stores or for purchase online.

Reverse osmosis filters are generally the best solution when they're practical because they address some other potential problems with your water. For example, municipal water sometimes contains fluoride, fertilizer and pesticide residues, pharmaceutical residues, volatile organic compounds, heavy metals, and, in some places, biological threats like amoebas and protozoa. You do not want to consume any of these, either.

In most places, if you ask them for it, your water company will provide you with a written analysis of your local water.

# SALT

- - - - - - - - - - - - - - - - - - - - - -

Partially refined sea salt is generally the best salt available. Sea salt naturally includes trace minerals that are important for your health, like magnesium, sulfur, manganese, boron, and silicon. Expect it to be gray, not white.

If you can't get good sea salt, it is too expensive in a particular context, or you are making a big batch of brine that will not be consumed directly, then look for

salt that contains only salt as an ingredient! Check the label. Kosher salt is often a good choice (but read the ingredients list).

Table salt often contains additives to prevent clumping. It may also contain additives to address some public health need, such as iodine to prevent goiter. These additives can add unpleasant tastes to foods and can impede your fermentation projects.

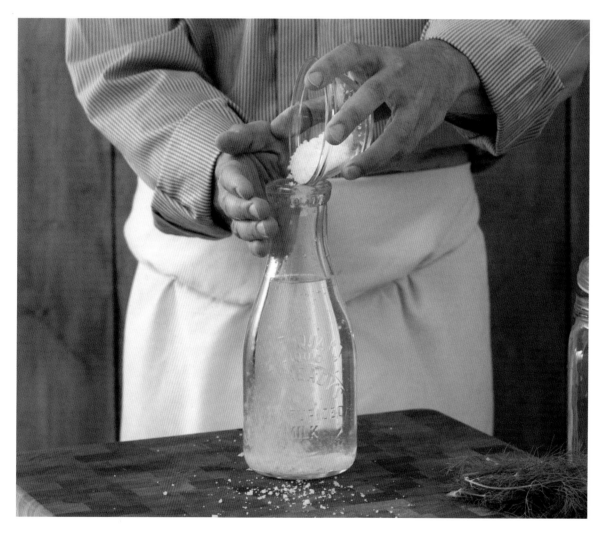

SALT IS AN ESSENTIAL INGREDIENT IN FERMENTATION RECIPES; HERE,
KOSHER SALT IS POURED INTO A CARAFE FOR MAKING BRINE.

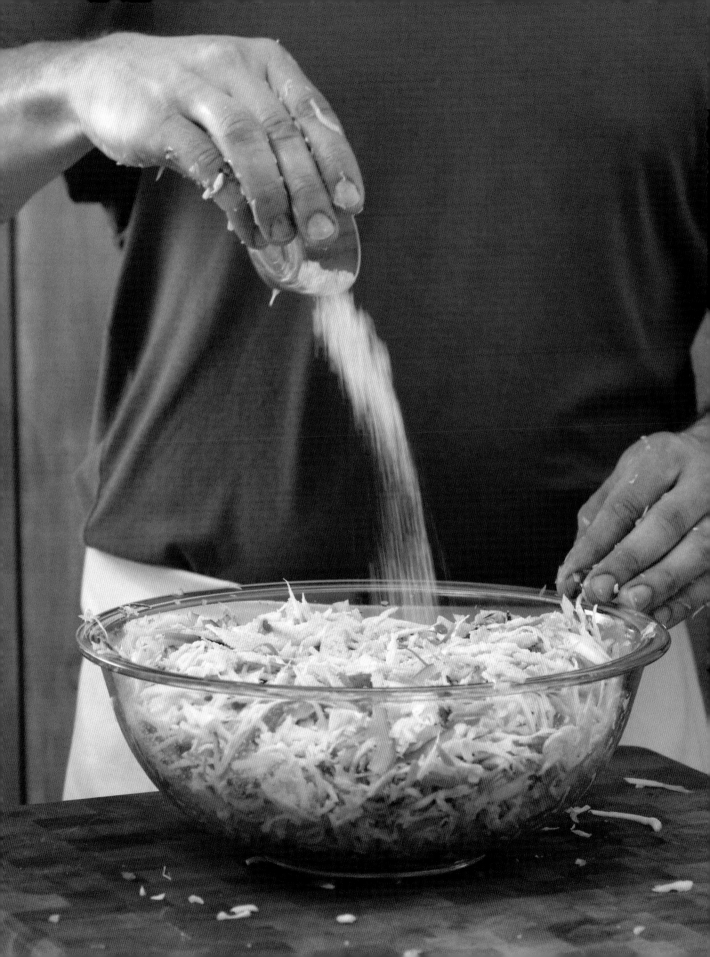

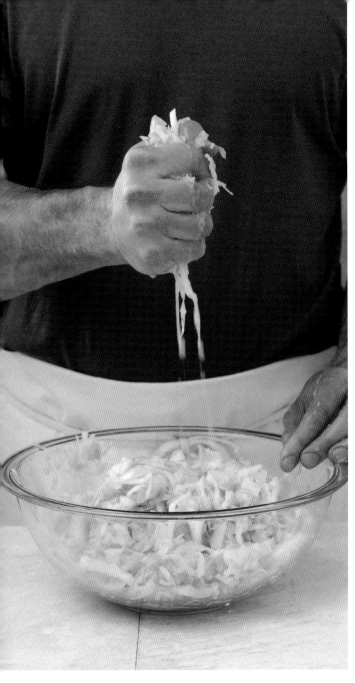

SQUEEZING LIQUID OUT OF A CABBAGE
AND SALT MIXTURE IN PREPARATION
FOR MAKING SAUERKRAUT (SEE RECIPE
ON PAGE 61)

# GETTING REAL ABOUT FOOD

Until a hundred or so years ago, most people in most parts of the world spent significant time pondering food, procuring food from nearby or known sources, and preparing food at home. Recently, we have spent less and less time on food. Over the course of the past century, we've gone from eating 98 percent of meals in our homes to 50 percent. And the food that we eat in our homes nowadays often comes in the form of frozen meals, "convenience" foods, soda, chips, and food-like substances that defy categorization. People in rich countries are not alone in this—the people of poorer countries have become eager consumers of soda, chips, and fast food and are squarely in the crosshairs of global food marketers.

Most snack foods, prepared foods, and restaurant foods in the United States, and in much of the world, are industrially produced. They are generally not environmentally sound because of the manufacture, processing, packaging, and transportation involved in their creation and delivery. Neither are they nutritionally sound: Their signature ingredients—high-fructose corn syrup, processed vegetable oils, white flour, flavoring chemicals, preservative chemicals, and so on—are used because they are cheap, addictive, and shelf stable, not because they are wholesome or nutritious in any way. In fact, many of these ingredients are harmful to us.

The best way for us to reverse this trend is simply to pay more attention to food. Every choice we make about food has an impact on the world. It also has an impact on us, for what we're putting into our bodies at that moment, for the habits we're forming for ourselves, and for the example that we're setting for others around us. Because you are reading this book, it's likely that you think about food more than most of the people you know—and it's likely that some of them look to you for guidance and inspiration about what and how to eat. (Some of them may have no choice!)

This is why it is important for us to make our own food.

On a broader level, thinking about food in a deep way can lead us to examine the politics and economics of food production and distribution. These issues are intertwined with some of the biggest problems of the day. It is easy to imagine how food politics might be related to famine and malnutrition, for instance. But there are many other problems in which food systems play a large role:

* chronic disease because of the way that diet affects health

* resource wars: today oil, soon water, because industrial food production relies on oil for fertilization, treatment, harvesting, and transportation, and on water for irrigation

* fragile financial markets and the complexities of globalization because the world is now one big, uneven market for commodity food

* use and misuse of technologies, including pesticides and weed killers, antibiotics, and genetically modified organisms

And so on.

## MAKING YOUR OWN FOOD

Every time you contemplate your next meal, you face choices.

**Where:** Do I eat at home or at a restaurant? When I'm eating with family or friends, do we make food and eat in our homes? Or do we go out?

**How:** Do I cook from scratch, completely or partially, or do I buy food that has been prepared ahead of time by someone else, using processes and ingredients that may or may not be what I would have preferred or expected?

**What:** Do I get my ingredients as directly as possible from their producers, or do I pay a commercial food aggregator (often a "supermarket") for the convenience of one-stop shopping?

Another consideration for most people is expense. How much does food cost where you live? How much of your income are you willing or able to spend on it? How much more would you spend to get food that tasted better? Or for food that you thought was better for you, or better for the world?

These are choices you make based on what is important to you.

When you decide to cook dinner for yourself and/or for others, what inspires you? How do you decide what you're going to cook? Once you have ideas, how do you decide where to get ingredients? Or do you go looking for ingredients first, and then decide what to make based on what you find? Are your ingredients generally raw materials like vegetables, meats, grains, fruits, herbs, and spices? Or are they more often things that have already been prepared or partially prepared, that may come in cans and boxes? Did you learn to cook from your family, from a cookbook, by watching television, or do you just "wing it"?

If you tell someone that you are cooking a meal "from scratch," what do your ingredients look like, and what processing might they have undergone before you got your hands on them?

## WHAT IS "FROM SCRATCH"?

To some people, cooking from scratch might mean making a casserole using a can of soup, a package of noodles, and some other things from packages and cans, then putting salad dressing from a bottle on a bag of mixed greens, and ending with a pie made with a store-bought crust. To others, cooking from scratch might mean raising a chicken, feeding the chicken, killing the chicken, making a soup from the chicken together with vegetables from the garden, grinding grains to make flour for bread or pasta, and so on. For most of us, it is probably somewhere between these two examples.

When I put more thought and attention into the process of choosing, preparing, and eating food, I feel more connected with that food and I feel better about it. Each of us has a different relationship with food, but often, the more of a role we had in its creation, the happier we are with it.

Preparing your own food increases your self-sufficiency. It also grants you greater control over what you are eating and enables you to make artistic and nutritional choices that would otherwise have been made by agents whose motivations may have more to do with their profit than with your health. And making food can be fun, and it can build family and community.

On a broader level, by choosing your food thoughtfully, you can register your vote against industrial food.

In modern societies, it is unrealistic to expect that every community will prepare all of its own food. But neither should we resign ourselves to eating 100 percent manufactured food. There is a broad middle ground, and we would do well to discover it, or to rediscover it.

So, how can you get started exploring new food ideas?

* One thing you can do is to buy less processed foods. Anything that comes in an opaque container, or in a container with a lot of writing on it, should be subject to scrutiny. If there is an ingredient list, does it match the picture on the box? If you had to make this thing yourself, could you? If you couldn't, or if you're not sure, you might think twice before buying it.

* Another thing you can do is to start a vegetable garden with your friends or family so that you can eat the freshest vegetables ever. You can even just grow some herbs on the windowsill, balcony, or driveway.

* Go to the farmers' market, and plan a meal around what you find there.

* Make a big batch of something from scratch. Arrange with your neighbors that they will do the same. Then have a big feast with them, or trade some of it with them, or freeze some of it.

Even if you can't do these things daily, keep them in mind.

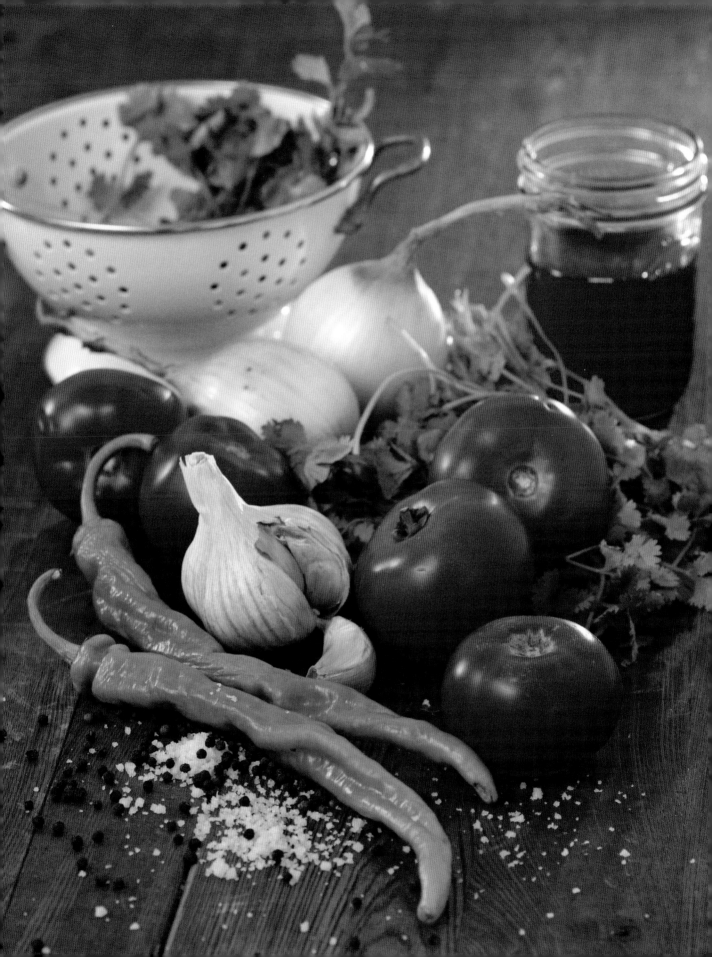

## FOOD AND POLITICS IN BOOKS AND MOVIES

For many years, there has been concern over some of the ugly implications of industrial food production.

★ More than 100 years ago, Upton Sinclair wrote a book called *The Jungle*. Though written as a novel, it was clearly intended to help create public outrage about the meat-packing industry, including the dangerous conditions that the workers had to endure, the greed and corruption of many of the managers, and the unhealthy product being sold to the public. The book succeeded in getting attention. Its descriptions of slaughterhouse conditions were proven to be accurate, and within two years of the book's publication, President Theodore Roosevelt, despite his strong antiregulatory orientation, was compelled to pass the Meat Inspection and Pure Food and Drug Acts, which paved the way for today's Food and Drug Administration (FDA).

★ Fifty years ago, Rachel Carson wrote *Silent Spring*, one of the most successful books to criticize the indiscriminate use of agricultural pesticides, particularly DDT. This book is widely credited with crystallizing the modern environmental movement in the United States and eventually led to the formation of the Environmental Protection Agency (EPA) and a ban on the use of DDT for agricultural purposes in the United States in 1973 (although American companies continued to export DDT to foreign markets into the 1980s, and it continues to be used in some poorer countries).

In recent years, there have been more and more books and films that have helped broaden awareness of the problems with industrial food:

★ In *Super Size Me,* filmmaker Morgan Spurlock investigates and illustrates the devastating health consequences of fast food by personally eating nothing but fast food for a month.

★ In her 2004 documentary *The Future of Food,* director Deborah Koons Garcia presents a disturbing picture of food technology trends and their impact on society and the environment.

★ Michael Pollan quips in his book *Food Rules* that we should not buy packaged foods containing more than five ingredients or foods that would baffle our great-grandmothers (food in a squeeze tube or spray can, for instance).

★ Robert Kenner's 2008 film *Food, Inc.* passes damning judgment on the industrial food production system, exposing how it feeds the wallets of food industry hegemons at the expense of ordinary, particularly rural and lower-income, people.

★ *The World According to Monsanto,* a 2008 film by Marie-Monique Robin, tells a disturbing story of collusion between industry and government to control food production at its very root: the farm.

★ Filmmaker Kristin Canty's 2011 film *Farmageddon* documents government regulators persecuting small farmers and ordinary citizens guilty of nothing more than trying to raise animals and produce and distribute food in nonindustrial ways. For example, a federal agency spent $1 million surveilling a sheep farm, and then confiscated and killed the animals in the name of a disease that never existed.

## THE INDIRECT COSTS OF INDUSTRIALIZED FOODS

----------------------------------------

One of the most important things about food that we ferment or prepare ourselves is precisely that we have done it ourselves; this food is more personal than food that has been created for us by strangers whom we never meet, that has visited factories and traveled nationally, or internationally, in trucks and cargo ships. We understand more about the history and context of homemade food, especially if we have bought the raw ingredients from people with whom we have a relationship.

Simon Fairlie, in his book *Meat: A Benign Extravagance*, presents a thorough critique of industrial animal farming and a brilliant exposition of the possibility for raising animals in a sustainable way. Many of his keenest observations apply equally to vegetable farming. He offers a succinct explication of the indirect costs of industrial foods:

" . . they are thickly implicated in a centralized distribution system which multiplies our energy expenditure at every opportunity and whose impacts include excessive packaging and refrigeration, waste, traffic congestion, road-building, noise, accidents, loss of local distinctiveness, exploitation and displacement of peasants, excessive immigration, urban slums, deforestation and habitat destruction, removal of biomass from third world countries, the undermining of local communities in the UK, the collapse of UK farming and the blood which is spilt over oil fields."

And while centralized distribution of food might seem, at first glance, to increase general access to food, in truth it does not. Because of the centralized structure of the industrial food system, food availability can be disrupted by terrorist attacks, energy crises, nuclear disasters, spikes in global commodity prices, and government overthrows. Any of these events can upset the delicate balance of the global food economy by cutting supply lines, increasing transportation costs, or pricing the world's poorest people out of the food market. Food security for large groups of people is tenuous.

This bleak list merely scratches the surface of the ills of industrial food. Other problems include toxic chemicals, unanswered questions about GMOs, decreasing biodiversity, the potential for large-scale food contamination (witness the ever-occurring problems with toxic strains of *E. coli*), waste disposal on large-scale animal farms, irrigation and water rights, indigenous land rights, and so on.

These are all reasons for us to understand local food where we live, develop relationships with food producers, and learn how to prepare and preserve our own food.

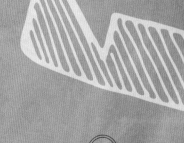

# REAL FOOD: I KNOW IT WHEN I SEE IT

Isn't it odd that we need to invent a term to describe the method of food production that was the only one available for most of human history?

Finding the right term for "not-industrial" food is tricky, for a couple of reasons.

First, the dividing lines are not clear. Some foods are more industrial, some are less, but most are somewhere in the middle. For example:

* Fruit can be grown with a lot of synthetic pesticides, less synthetic pesticides, and/or pesticides made from natural sources that are nonetheless toxic.

* "Free range" chickens must have outdoor areas available to them, but these areas may be tiny, and the chickens are not necessarily encouraged to visit them, so they may never go outdoors. The same chickens may be fed 100 percent vegetarian diets, which sounds great, except when you realize that until recently, there were no vegetarian chickens— chickens love eating worms and bugs.

* Fields can be worked using great big powered machines, small machines, draft animals, or hand tools. Different people may have different feelings about which of these are or are not "industrial."

Second, many of the words that have been used to describe not-industrial foods have taken on meanings that are either too narrow or too broad.

* "Organic" used to be a general indicator of "not-industrial," but it has recently taken on specific, legal meanings.

* "Natural" is another word that could be the opposite of "industrial;" however in many places, there are no regulations, or confusing regulations, around its use. Since marketers became fond of it, it has become more or less meaningless.

* "Sustainable" has the right feeling to it, but it is quickly becoming a marketing buzzword, too.

* The word "conventional," despite its typical connotations of "traditional" and "old-fashioned," has come to mean the opposite of these; it is used to denote food that has been produced using chemicals and modern industrial methods. These so-called conventions are very new and were certainly not norms 100 years ago.

Where does that leave us?

The term "slow food" is popular. In fact, Slow Food is the name of an organization that was created to reverse the trend toward industrialized food. Its name was chosen to suggest the opposite of "fast food." By their own report, "Slow Food is a global, grassroots organization with supporters in 150 countries around the world who are linking the pleasure of good food with a commitment to their community and the environment." But because the term "slow food" is associated with a specific organization, it is not ideal for general use.

"Real food" may be the best term that has emerged in the past several years. It's not clear who coined it, or even when, and it does not have specific associations like "slow food" does.

What exactly is "real food"? U.S. Supreme Court Justice Potter Stewart memorably said about pornography that it is difficult to define, but "I know it when I see it." The situation is the same, I think, with real food. Each of us knows it when we see it, even though we may disagree on some of the details.

So for now, "real food" is a good label.

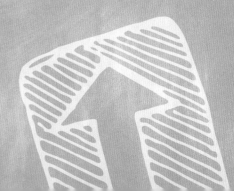

# REAL FOOD, REAL MISSION

The arguments about food and politics can be quite abstract. How can we think of it in more personal terms?

★ By procuring our own ingredients and preparing our own food, we can reground ourselves (literally, if we eat from our own gardens!).

★ Fermenting affords us a unique way to preserve and enhance our own foods without the need for chemicals or even fossil fuel–fed heating or cooling systems.

★ Fermenting enhances foods' vitamin and enzyme contents, increases mineral bioavailability, and benefits our digestion, thus fortifying the physical body.

★ The relative reliability of the lacto-fermentation process can give us a feeling of control and agency in a universe that has become increasingly frustrating: an anchor in a stormy sea. *Lactobacillus* is a constant friend, even when others are fickle.

★ On an even more spiritual level, lacto-fermentation is a sort of alchemy or magic, transforming workaday, gas-inducing raw cabbage into extraordinary sauerkraut and turning garden-variety lemons into exotic delicacies.

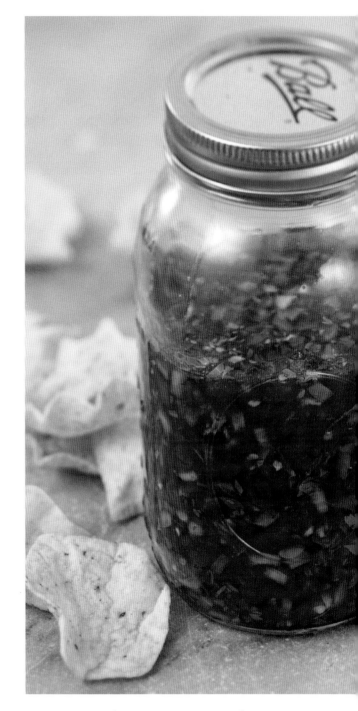

PICO DE GALLO (SEE RECIPE ON PAGE 122)

# CHAPTER 3

# SAUERKRAUT

SAUERKRAUT IS A FOOD whose salient ingredient is lacto-fermented cabbage—green, red, savoy, or napa.

Sauerkraut has a colorful history. It has existed in one form or another, by one name or another, for at least several thousand years. Evidence has been found of sauerkraut in the diets of the workers building the Great Wall of China; Pliny wrote of sauerkraut in ancient Rome; fermented cabbage has been a mainstay of cold-weather European diets since at least the Middle Ages; and sailors have carried it on ships to ward off scurvy, which it can do because of its high vitamin C content.

AS A FIRST FERMENTATION PROJECT, sauerkraut is ideal. It is simple and relatively quick to make, has a high success rate, and is delicious. Sauerkraut can be eaten on its own, of course, but it can also be eaten on a sandwich, in a soup or stew, with meat or fish, with eggs, in a dumpling, or however you like.

Its appeal is international. Kimchi—a sauerkraut variant that includes ginger, garlic, onions, and, often, spicy red pepper and other seasonings—is the uncontested national dish of Korea. It is often eaten for three meals a day, as a side dish, and also in stews, stir-fries, fried rice, soup, and so on. *Choucroute garnie*, which I think of as "the queen of sauerkraut dishes," is a casserole of pork, sausages, potatoes, juniper berries, Riesling, and, of course, sauerkraut that is a favorite in the Alsace region of France. Sauerkraut also figures prominently in all the food cultures of central Europe as well as all the cultures they have influenced.

## WHY YOU MUST READ THIS CHAPTER

Even if you don't like sauerkraut, please read this chapter anyway. The issues that come up while making sauerkraut are the same issues that come up while making other fermented vegetables and fruits. Thus, sauerkraut is a great jumping-off point and an excellent template for further fermenting adventures. And maybe if you made your own sauerkraut you would like it!

Important parts of the sauerkraut-making process that apply to other fermenting projects include the following:

* selecting raw materials and equipment

* using a knife and cutting board

* measuring and weighing ingredients

* mixing the vegetables with salt

* deciding whether to add a fermentation starter

* packing the product tightly in a fermenting jar

* testing it for readiness

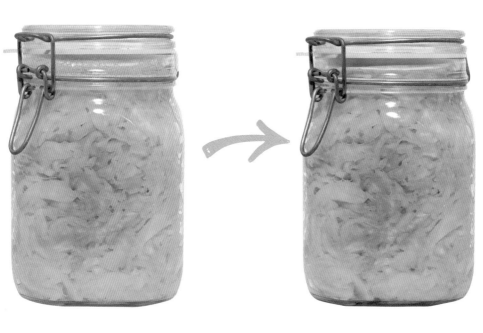

RED CABBAGE SAURKRAUT
AT 5 DAYS

RED CABBAGE SAURKRAUT
AT 10 DAYS

THE EVOLUTION OF SAUERKRAUT

GREEN CABBAGE SAURKRAUT
AT 5 DAYS

GREEN CABBAGE SAURKRAUT
AT 10 DAYS

# BASIC SAUERKRAUT

In its basic form, sauerkraut contains only two ingredients: cabbage and salt. The recipe can be varied by adding other vegetables or seasonings. By eating it young or letting it ferment for a longer time, you can choose between crunchy, slightly sour cabbage; epic, Wagnerian SAUERKRAUT; or anything in between.

## INGREDIENTS

2 pounds (900 g) cabbage (green and red cabbage work best for this simple sauerkraut recipe)

4 teaspoons (20 g) sea salt

## EQUIPMENT

Large cutting board (wood is ideal)

Large knife (a chef's knife is ideal)

Large mixing bowl

1-quart (950-ml) mason jar, or similar glass jar with a tight-fitting lid

*Recipe continued on page 62*

**Yield: 1 quart (950 ml)**

**Prep time: 10 minutes**

**Total time: 4 days–4 weeks**

## WEIGHING

If your cabbage is not exactly 2 pounds (900 g), use approximately 2 teaspoons (10 g) of sea salt per pound (450 g) of cabbage. Alternatively, you can use 2 percent salt by weight.

For best results, weigh your cabbage *after* you have removed its outer leaves and core.

## JARS

For each pound (450 g) of cabbage you use, you will need 16 ounces (475 ml) of jar capacity, or a bit more. Depending on the size of your jars, you can use a small jar to help pack the sauerkraut into the bigger jars (in step 10).

## PREPARATION

1　Peel off the outer leaves of the cabbage and discard them (a). (Note: This is particularly important if your cabbage is not organically grown. For more on choosing ingredients, see chapter 2.)

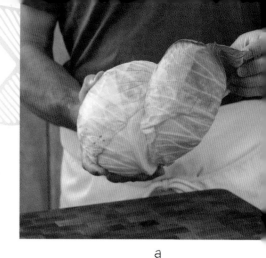

a

2　If you are working with a whole cabbage, cut it in half, from the south pole to the north pole (b).

3　Cut each half once more, along the north-south axis, so that the whole cabbage is now in four pieces (c).

4　*Optional:* Remove some of the core of the cabbage by cutting diagonally into each quarter (d).

5　With its south pole facing you, lay a quarter of the cabbage on your cutting board, and slice it as finely or as coarsely as you like (e). More finely cut cabbage will ferment more quickly and will become a softer kraut. Coarser cut cabbage will lead to a crunchier product. Be careful of your fingers!

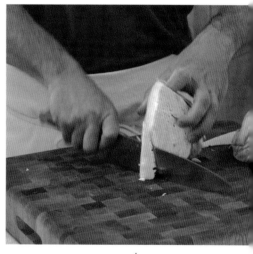

d

6　When it becomes awkward to slice, turn or flip the cabbage quarter in whatever way is convenient to make it more stable on the cutting board and easier to cut.

7　If you prefer, use a food processor with a "slice" wheel to shred your cabbage (f). You could also use a deli-style meat slicer, a box grater, or a purpose-built *Krauthobel*.

8　Slice the rest of the cabbage in this manner. When you are done, put it all in the mixing bowl and add the salt (g).

9　With clean hands, *firmly* massage the mixture of cabbage and salt until you are able to squeeze liquid out of the cabbage (h). Depending on how fresh the cabbage is, how much cabbage you have, and how hard you are squeezing, this may take anywhere from 1 to 10 minutes. You will develop a feel for it after you have done it a few times.

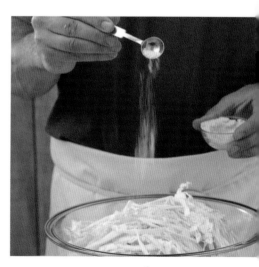

g

10　Pack the mixture into a jar or jars (i). Using an appropriately sized implement, such as a small jar or potato masher, push down as hard as you can to get rid of as many air bubbles as possible, so that the liquid rises above the top of the cabbage. Ensure that there is at least 1 inch (2.5 cm) of space between the top of the cabbage and the mouth of the jar, because the cabbage will expand as it ferments.

11　Close the lid of the jar and place it in a cool, dark place, if possible (between 50°F and 75°F [10°C and 25°C]).

*Recipe continued on page 64*

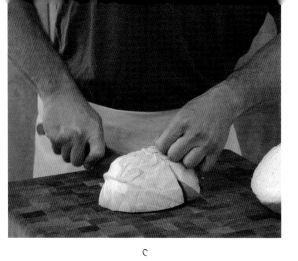

b

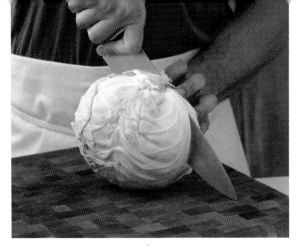

c

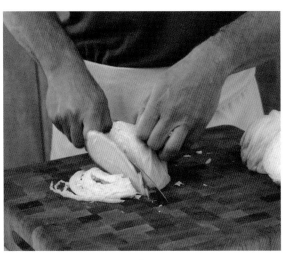

e

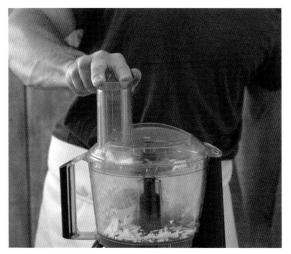

f (optional)

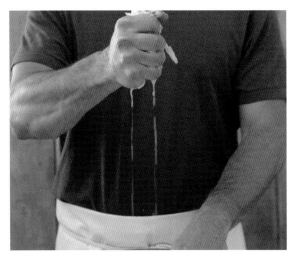

h

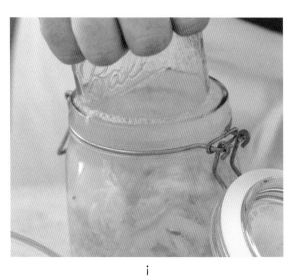

i

## FERMENTATION PROCESS

Check on your sauerkraut every day or two. Open the jar, smell it, taste it with a clean fork, and pack the sauerkraut back down until the liquid rises above it. After a few days, it should get bubbly. After a few more days, it should start to smell and taste sour.

You can eat it any time you want, or you can put it the refrigerator to arrest its progress. Young sauerkraut is crunchier; older sauerkraut has a stronger flavor.

For maximum digestive and nutritive benefits, eat your sauerkraut raw (i.e., do not heat it beyond about 115°F [46°C]). However, if digestive and nutritive benefits are not your main goals, there's no shame in cooking your sauerkraut. In fact, old sauerkraut that has become soggy and very sour may taste best cooked.

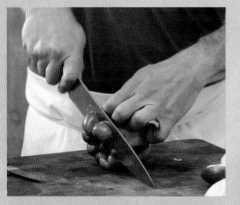

a

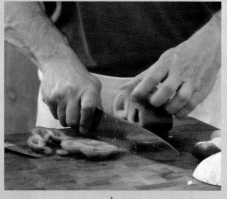

b

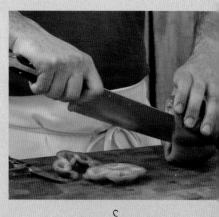

c

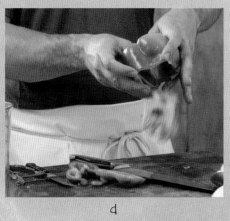

d

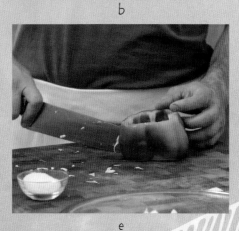

e

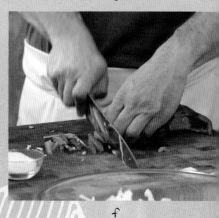

f

This is a great process for cutting a bell pepper. It's particularly useful when readying bell peppers for fermentation, as in the recipe on page 79 for Fermented Carolina-Style Slaw.

## CUTTING A BELL PEPPER

1   Cut both top and bottom off the pepper (a), (b).

2   Run your knife around the inside of the pepper (c).

3   Put down your knife, and eject the seeds and core of the pepper by pushing with your thumbs (d).

4   Cut the pepper vertically (e) and lay it flat (f), or cut it into rings, or cut it however you want. Use the end pieces, too, if you like.

# CHAPTER 4

# BEYOND BASIC SAUERKRAUT: LACTO-FERMENTED VEGETABLES

SAUERKRAUT, MADE WITH CABBAGE AND SALT, is the archetype of fermented vegetables. But cabbage is not the only vegetable that can be fermented, and salt is not the only seasoning that can be added to fermented vegetables. You can ferment other vegetables along with cabbage, without changing the proportion of vegetable to salt. You can ferment a vegetable mix containing little or no cabbage.

You can even throw in some fruit. Other vegetables and fruit may be trickier to ferment than cabbage, but you can do things to improve your chances of success. You can also make fermented foods with little or no salt if you like; in this case, you may need to use some tricks to help ensure that the right bacteria prevail.

This chapter answers many of the questions that may come up when fermenting vegetables.

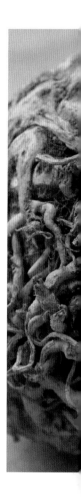

# WHICH VEGETABLES (AND/OR FRUIT) SHOULD I USE?

Some vegetables, like cabbage, ferment easily, while others require extra attention, guidance, and/or coercion.

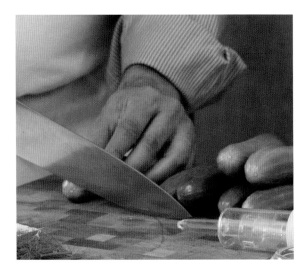

### GOOD FERMENTERS

The best fermenting vegetables are from the family *Brassicaceae*, also known as cruciferous vegetables. These include cabbage, turnips, kohlrabi, and radishes. They have a firm texture and relatively low sugar content.

### OKAY FERMENTERS

Vegetables like onions, carrots, and celery root do well when mingled with good fermenters. If you seek to ferment them on their own, you might want to use a starter (see page 72).

### TEMPERAMENTAL FERMENTERS

When most people think of pickles and pickling, they think of cucumbers. Interestingly, fermenting cucumbers can be tricky. Fermented cucumbers can succumb to "hollow pickle syndrome," wherein the inside of the pickle disintegrates; this is often accompanied by general softness of the pickle. Likewise, summer squashes and bell peppers can become disconcertingly soft (ripe bell peppers are worse than green ones). These problems come from the work of enzymes on the relatively weak physical structure of these vegetables.

With vegetables that don't ferment very well, consider using a starter, using a generous concentration of salt, and even seeking additional insurance (see page 73). Cutting off the blossom ends of these vegetables mitigates some of the enzyme issues, too (see chapter 1).

Beets, parsnips, apples, pears, and other sweet fruit, because of their higher sugar content, tend to attract yeasts that can cause the fermentation to veer off in the direction of alcohol generation. This is great if you are trying to make an alcoholic beverage, but if you are trying to make lacto-fermented vegetables and fruit, it is not what you want. If you combine these sweet vegetables and fruits with well-behaved ones like cabbage and turnips, you will generally get the results you expect i.e. lacto-fermentation. Sweet vegetables and fruit can be lacto-fermented on their own with the use of a starter.

### VEGETABLES TO AVOID

Raw potatoes contain compounds called glycoalkaloids, which are neurotoxic (poisonous to your brain and your nervous system). So potatoes are not good candidates for raw fermenting—or raw anything, for that matter.

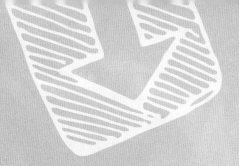

## TROUBLESHOOTING: FERMENTATION GONE WRONG

What can go wrong with a vegetable ferment, and how can I fix it?

**If it tastes too salty:** Add water judiciously, stir the whole thing up, possibly drain out some of the liquid, and give everything some time to rebalance.

**If the top of the batch of vegetables has dried up:** It may be possible to revive the batch by stirring it up (submerging the dry part at the top), and then adding some water or brine.

**If the vegetables have become too soft or mushy:** You cannot reverse this, but if they are just a little soft or mushy, they may be used in a soup or a stew, where vegetables go to become soft and mushy anyway. They are best added at the last minute, or even after the dish has started to cool, so that they don't cook for a long time and become even more soft and mushy, and also so that their beneficial microbes and nutrients aren't all destroyed by heat.

If they became too soft sooner than you hoped, there are measures you can take in the future to improve the texture. These measures include using more salt, using a starter, or adding something else, like grape leaves, for the specific purpose of decreasing mushiness (see page 73 for more on fermenting "insurance").

**If the vegetables have become slimy, if there is visible fuzz or significant mold growing on top, or if they smell bad or of alcohol:** This indicates that the fermentation did not go as planned, probably having been hijacked by molds or yeasts or both. It won't taste good, it won't have good texture, and eating it could be risky. Send it to the compost heap!

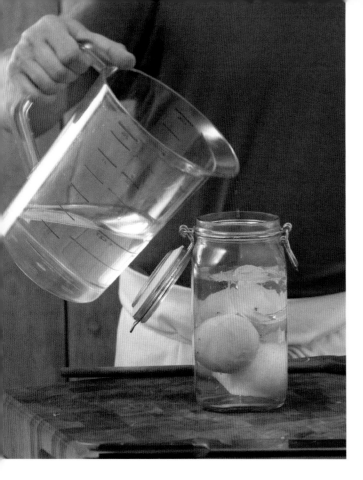

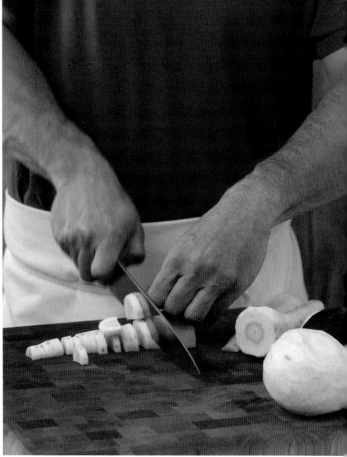

# HOW SHOULD I CUT THE VEGETABLES? OR SHOULD I?

Vegetables can be left whole, sliced, shredded, or cut into matchsticks or pretty much any which way. Some key considerations:

★ Thicker things take longer to ferment and can have more problems. With some vegetables this is an issue, while with others it is not. Sauerkraut and kimchi can be made with whole or quartered cabbages, and turnips can be fermented whole without concern. On the other hand, fermenting large cucumbers or squash can be tricky, for the reasons outlined on page 68.

★ Fibrous vegetables are best cut across the fibers, rather than parallel to them. This will make them more pleasant to eat. Parsnips, for instance, should be cut into coins rather than sticks.

★ For culinary and aesthetic reasons, you may want to cut all of the components of a dish to the same general size and shape. For instance, if you are making a coleslaw-style vegetable mix, you might aim to cut or shred the cabbage, carrot, onion, and pepper similarly. For a kimchi mix, you might try to cut everything into 1-inch (2.5 cm) lengths or squares.

★ You may also choose to create a mixture of different shapes and sizes. A Brussels sprout or turnip or two in a jar of sauerkraut can add a nice surprise.

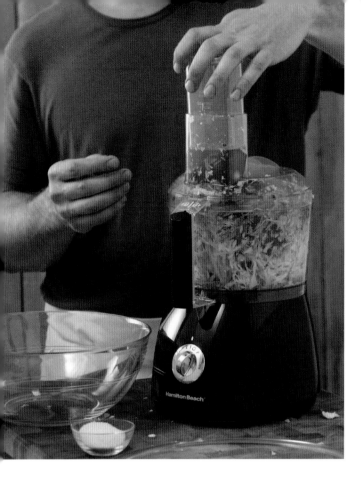
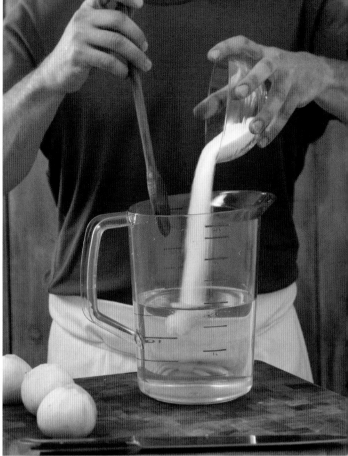

# WILL I NEED TO ADD MORE LIQUID TO SUBMERGE EVERYTHING?

With certain vegetables, certain cuts, and the right amount of salt, adding liquid may not be necessary. But if you seek to ferment whole vegetables on their own, such as a barrel of cabbages, a bucket of cucumbers, or a jar of radishes, you will need to submerge them in brine.

Here's how to make brine:

1 tablespoon (15 g) salt (see page 48) per cup (250 ml) of water

This brine has a concentration of 6 percent salt by weight and is a good starting point. If you use this to ferment vegetables and the result is too salty, add a splash more water and let it sit for a bit; if the result is too mushy, chalk one up to experience, and use more salt, a starter, or some additional insurance (see page 73) next time.

# DO I NEED TO PEEL EVERYTHING BEFOREHAND?

Organic whole vegetables may be peeled or not, as you like. If not peeled, they can be scrubbed clean with a vegetable brush; soap is not needed. Nonorganic vegetables should always be peeled to get rid of as much of the pesticide residue as possible; nonorganic leafy vegetables should have their outer leaves removed.

# WHICH STARTER SHOULD I USE, IF ANY?

A starter is a collection of microbes that you add to your food to encourage it to ferment in the way that you want.

Fermentation projects based on well-behaved fermenters and salt do not generally require a starter because they naturally tend to attract the right sorts of microbes. Projects based on more troublesome vegetables and fruits, or lower than usual amounts of salt, on the other hand, can benefit from a nudge (or a shove) in the right direction.

You have three options (at least) for fermented vegetable starters:

**Liquid from a previous batch of homemade sauerkraut or other fermented vegetables (not too young and not too old—say, between 4 days and 4 weeks):** This starter is often a good choice. It is easy to make, and its freshness is known. It tends to impart a fermented vegetable flavor when added; in many cases (when making fermented vegetables, for instance), this is not a problem.

**Live dairy whey from yogurt, kefir, or clabbered raw milk (the younger the better):** This is a good, powerful starter that is easy to make. To make yogurt whey, put yogurt in cheesecloth; the liquid that drips out is whey. (See recipe on page 102.) Whey can impart a slight milky taste or texture, even when strained carefully. Because it is a dairy product, vegans, kosher eaters, and those with sensitivity to casein or acute sensitivity to lactose should be aware of this.

**Purpose-made vegetable fermentation starter culture:** Powdered starter cultures are sold in envelopes. They should be kept cool until used, and it is important to pay attention to their expiration dates. A purpose-made starter, assuming it has been transported and stored properly, can produce excellent, consistent results without any stray flavors. However, these starters do cost money, and purists might object to using these packaged goods. They sometimes contain dairy.

# DO I WANT ADDITIONAL FERMENTING INSURANCE?

As I noted previously, cucumber pickles and summer squash have a tendency to digest themselves. (This self-digestion is called autolysis.) Even a recipe that works most of the time, in most places, might not turn out as you had hoped, depending on the ingredients you are using, the temperature and humidity, the ambient bacteria where you are, or just plain bad luck.

Beyond using a starter, there are a few things you can do to further improve your odds of success, especially with cucumbers:

★ You can add some vinegar to immediately increase acidity. Boiled red wine vinegar and cider vinegar are good options because of the tannins they contain (see the next item); distilled white vinegar works well, too. Raw wine or cider vinegar may not work as well because they contain their own set of microbes that are not really the ones you want and that could potentially take over your pickles. If you'd like to use wine or cider vinegar, boil it first, and then let it cool.

★ For centuries, people have been adding grape leaves, oak leaves, bay leaves, and other tannic leaves to cucumber pickles in order to keep them crunchy. As we now know, tannins inhibit cucumbers' naturally occurring pectinase and cellulase enzymes that would otherwise cause the cucumbers to digest themselves. Grape skins contain tannins, too, so red wine vinegar can be a double help. Other good sources of tannins include apple cider vinegar, cloves, tarragon, cumin, thyme, vanilla, and cinnamon—some of which are found in pickling spice mixes (I don't think this is a coincidence). Finally, black tea, loose or in tea bags, contains tannins and can give your pickles a little caffeine kick!

★ A small amount (concentrations of up to 0.5 percent) of calcium chloride ("cackle") may be added to brine for cucumber pickles to act as an enzyme inhibitor. Calcium chloride is also used when curing olives. If you go this route, be sure to get food-grade calcium chloride, not the kind that you spread on sidewalks to melt ice!

★ Aluminum sulfate ("alum") is also sometimes used in pickle making. It is a common ingredient in baking powder. Unfortunately, it is a neurotoxin and should be shunned.

# WHICH SEASONINGS SHOULD I ADD?

When deciding how to season your fermented vegetables, you have a lot of leeway. Beyond salt, which serves a specific function in the fermentation process, you can add pretty much whatever seasonings you like, in whatever amounts you like. I encourage you to experiment. It's generally fine to add seasonings at or near the end of the fermentation process. You can feel free to make lots of little containers of fermented vegetables, season each of them differently, taste them, and pick some favorites. And do not fear failure; there are always more vegetables to be fermented.

Here are a few ideas about herbs, spices, and flavorings to get you started:

★ Salt, probably. If you want to use less than a typical amount of salt, you may want to use more starter to ensure a good microbial balance.

★ Caraway seeds and juniper berries are traditional in European sauerkrauts; cumin, fennel, anise, and other seeds provide interesting variations, as does schizandra.

* Dill is a classic seasoning for sour pickles; fennel and lovage suggest themselves as possibilities. Garlic and celery seed work well, too.

* A traditional "pickling spice" mix might contain red and black pepper, coriander, cumin, ginger, allspice, cinnamon, bay leaf, mustard seed, clove, and turmeric.

* Asian sauerkrauts, like kimchi, start with napa cabbage, daikon, or mustard greens; they often include ginger, garlic, onion, and hot red pepper; turmeric, galangal, and burdock are all welcome additions.

* South American sauerkrauts may include cabbage, red onion, carrot, oregano, and dried or fresh chile pepper; think about other members of the mint family, and/or cilantro. It's great to add olive oil when you're about to serve it.

* Carolina-style coleslaw, which was almost certainly fermented rather than vinegared a few generations ago, starts with cabbage, onion, green bell pepper, shredded carrot, mustard, and celery seed or root. Again, oil can be added when it's ready to be served.

* In addition to everything already mentioned, consider mace, thyme, cardamom, and shallot.

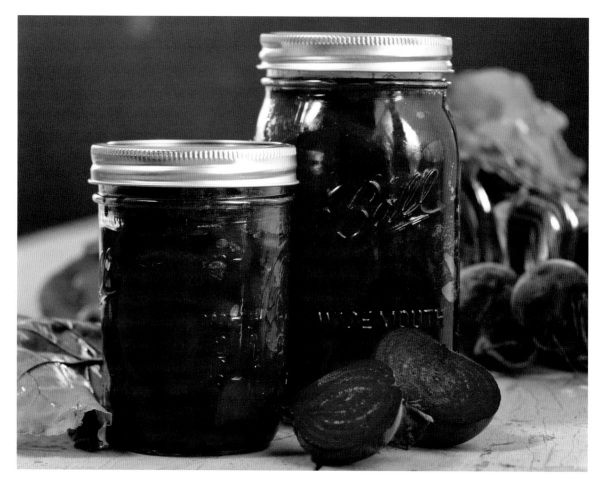

CELERY ROOT

# LACTO-FERMENTED VEGETABLES

This recipe is very similar to the recipe for Basic Sauerkraut on page 61. Consider reading that one first for an in-depth introduction!

## INGREDIENTS

2 pounds (900 g) cabbage, turnips, radishes, kohlrabi, celery root, and/or other vegetables, as desired

4 teaspoons (20 g) sea salt

Seasonings, as desired

## EQUIPMENT

Large cutting board (wood is ideal)

Large knife (a chef's knife is ideal)

Large mixing bowl

1-quart (950 ml) mason jar, or similar glass jar with a tight-fitting lidd

*Recipe continued on page 76*

**Yield: 1 quart (950 ml)**

**Prep time: 10 minutes**

**Total time: 4 days–4 weeks**

## PREPARATION

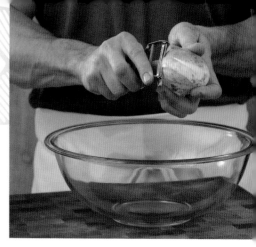

a

1   Peel, shred, core, seed, chop, and/or slice your vegetables, as desired. Carrots, turnips, beets, and the like may be peeled (a) (see page 72), and they may be shredded or cut (b).

2   Weigh all of the vegetables together, after you have peeled, cored, and otherwise prepped them.

3   Measure 2 teaspoons (10 g) of sea salt per pound (450 g) of vegetables (or 2 percent salt by weight).

4   Combine the vegetables and the salt in the mixing bowl (c).

5   Massage them together forcefully with your hands, for a minute or two (d).

6   Pack the vegetables into the jar with your hands as tightly as possible (e).

7   Use a smaller jar, a bottle, a potato masher, or some other rigid object to pack the vegetables even more tightly into the jar. Ideally, when you push down, liquid will rise above the tops of the vegetables (f). Close the jar tightly.

8   Open the jar and pack its contents down a few times over the next couple of days.

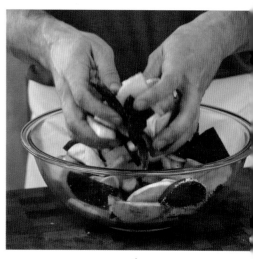

d

Turnips and beets, cut into rounds or matchsticks, are a great combination (g). They get tender and juicy after several days. Add parsnips, too, cut into rounds, if you like (h).

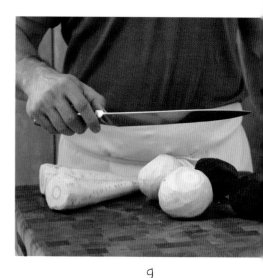

g

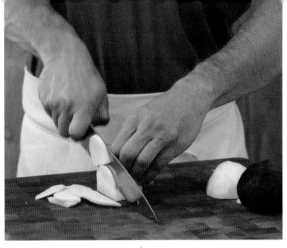

b

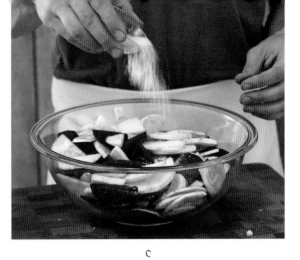

c

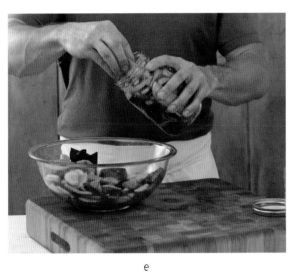

e

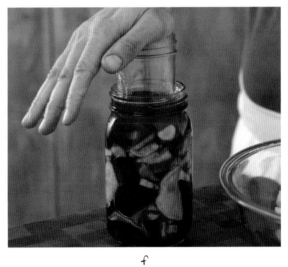

f

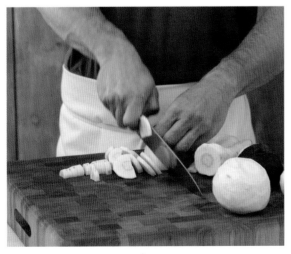

h

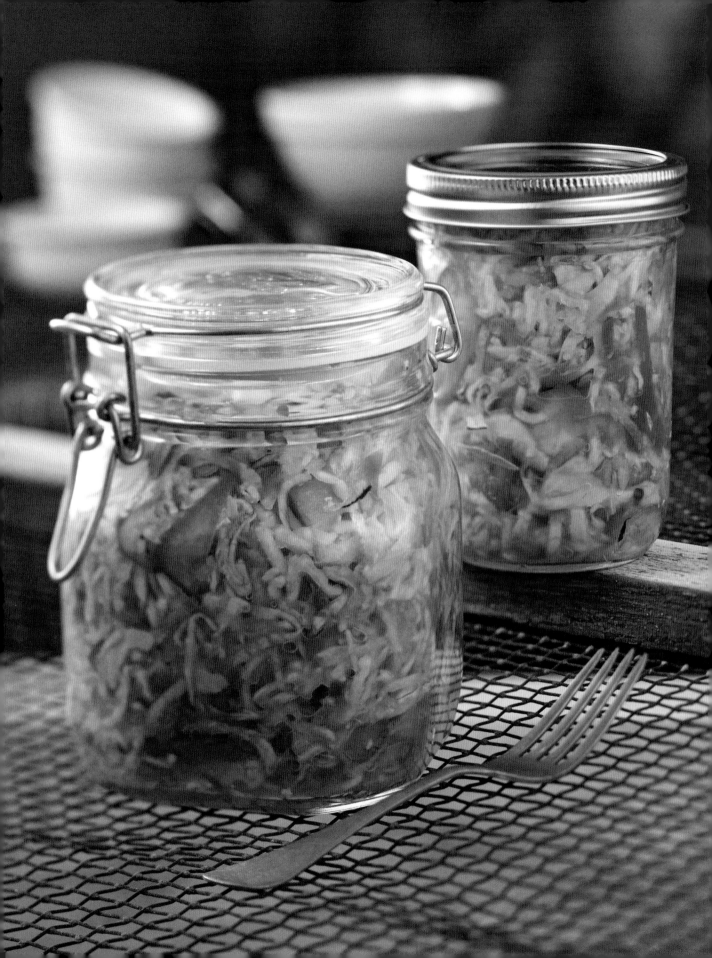

# FERMENTED CAROLINA-STYLE SLAW

Carolina-style slaw is a type of coleslaw that is traditional in the southeastern United States. The dressing for this coleslaw is similar to a vinaigrette salad dressing and does not contain mayonnaise or sour cream like some other sorts of coleslaw. I generally prefer Carolina-style coleslaw to the creamy kind. Especially if I'm having barbecued meats, for instance, or other heavy or fatty foods, a creamy slaw is "too much of the same"—I'm happier with a clean, crisp, and sour slaw.

It's clear to me that today's Carolina slaw, soured with vinegar, is a re-creation of the slaws of yesteryear, which must have been fermented—soured via bacterial action—because that was how one kept cabbage. I would like to bring back this fermented slaw. The big benefit, besides taste and texture, is that the fermentation process makes everything easier to digest—both the cabbage and whatever it's accompanying.

The same recipe can be made with whatever vegetables you like, selected according to the criteria outlined earlier in this chapter and in chapter 2. Cabbage relatives are good choices. Some possibilities include broccoli, cauliflower, Brussels sprouts, and shredded turnip. Or you could replace all the cabbage with celery root if you wanted to.

## INGREDIENTS

1 pound (450 g) green cabbage

1 large onion (red, yellow, or white)

1 large green bell pepper

1 large carrot

$\frac{1}{2}$ apple (optional)

$\frac{1}{4}$ pound (115 g) celery root, or 1 teaspoon celery seed

4 teaspoons (20 g) sea salt

$\frac{1}{4}$ cup (80 g) honey (or less, if you have included an apple)

6 tablespoons (90 ml) oil (a mixture of sesame, coconut, and olive oils works well)

2 teaspoons dry mustard

1 piece ($\frac{1}{3}$ inch, or 8 mm) gingerroot, peeled and grated (optional)

Freshly ground black pepper

**Yield: 1 quart (950 ml), or 2 pounds (900 g)**

**Prep time: 20 minutes**

**Total time: 4–7 days**

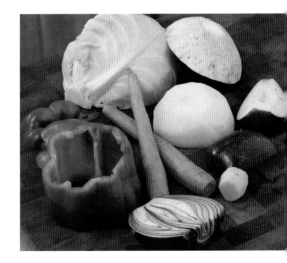

*Recipe continued on page 80*

**Fermented Carolina-Style Slaw continued**

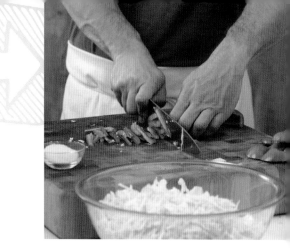

## EQUIPMENT

Large cutting board (wood is ideal)

Large knife (a chef's knife is ideal)

Large mixing bowl

2 mason jars (1 pint, or 475 ml each) or similar glass jars with tight-fitting lids

Colander or strainer

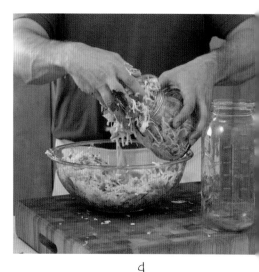

a

## PREPARATION

1 Thinly slice the cabbage, onion, and bell pepper (a). (For tips on how to cut a bell pepper, see page 65.)

2 Grate or shred the carrot, apple, if using, and celery root, if using (b).

3 Ferment the vegetable mixture with the salt using the recipe for Lacto-Fermented Vegetables on page 75, to the desired degree of sourness (c), (d), (e). Four to seven days is probably about right.

4 Once the vegetables are fermented, drain them in a colander set over a mixing bowl, and press the liquid out with your hands, reserving the liquid.

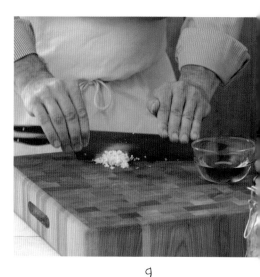

d

5 Combine ¹/₂ cup (120 ml) of the liquid with the honey, oil, dry mustard, and ginger, and mix well with a fork, whisk, or blender (f), (g). Pour the dressing mixture and combine (h). Add salt and pepper as needed. Add more of the reserved liquid if you want more sourness. Refrigerate.

Save any leftover fermentation liquid to use as a starter for your next project. Or mix it with oil and spices to use as a salad dressing. Or drink it in the morning as a digestive tonic!

g

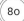

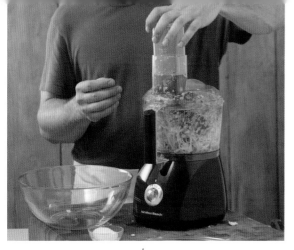

b

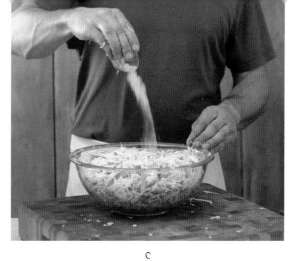

c

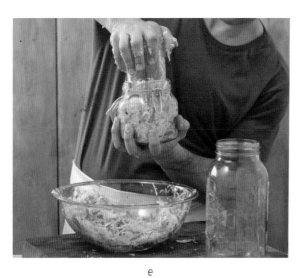

e

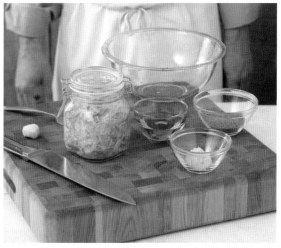

f

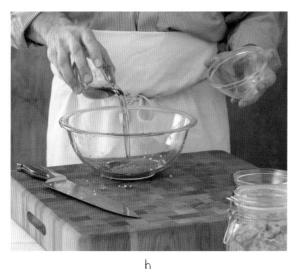

h

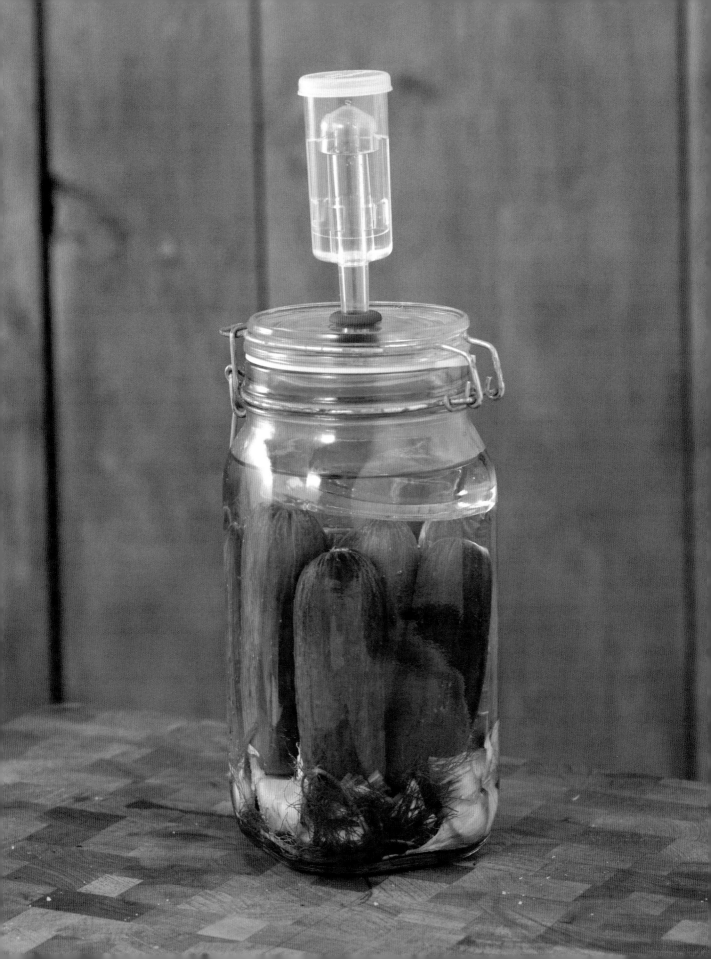

# CUCUMBER PICKLES

Pickled cucumbers, or simply "pickles," are another quintessential fermented food. The first record of pickles comes from ancient Mesopotamia. Such diverse historical figures as Aristotle, Julius Caesar, Shakespeare, Amerigo Vespucci, and Thomas Jefferson are reported to have been fond of pickles. Indeed, Amerigo Vespucci, after whom America was named, was a pickle vendor before he became a world explorer.

Pickles play a significant role in the food culture of many countries, from North America through Europe and into the Middle East.

## INGREDIENTS

3 or 4 pounds (1.5 or 2 kg) small, thick-skinned cucumbers

2 quarts (2 L) chlorine-free water

½ cup (115 g) sea salt

Up to 1 cup (250 ml) whey or 1 pint (475 ml) sauerkraut juice, or starter powder from an envelope (optional)

Seasonings: generous amounts of whole garlic, bay leaf, etc. (optional)

A few fresh grape or oak leaves, or a couple of black tea bags, for their tannins (optional)

Red wine vinegar or apple cider vinegar, boiled and cooled to replace up to half of the water (optional)

**Yield: 3–4 pounds (1.5–2 kg)**

**Prep time: 10 minutes**

**Total time: 3 days–2 weeks**

*Recipe continued on page 84*

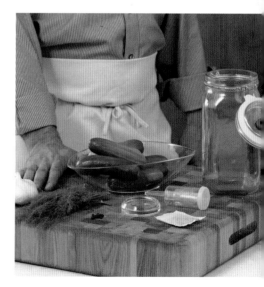

Cucumber Pickles continued

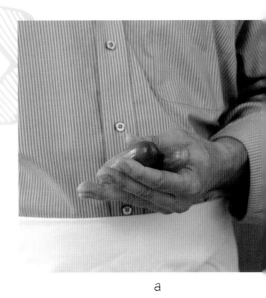

a

## EQUIPMENT

Knife

Cutting board (wood is ideal)

1-gallon (4-L) pitcher

½-gallon (2-L) mason jar, a Pickl-It, a Harsch crock, or a plain glazed (lead-free) ceramic crock

Something to hold the cucumbers under the brine, like a small clean plate or saucer that fits inside the jar or crock (if needed)

Clean dishtowel or cloth to cover the top of the jar or crock along with a rubber band (if needed)

## PREPARATION

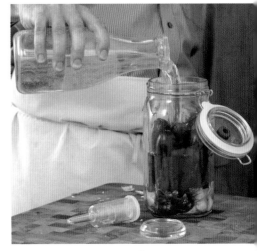

d

1   If your cucumbers are at all soft, if you bought them at the store, and/or if you suspect that they might have been picked a while ago, you can perk them up by soaking them in ice water (a).

2   Trim the blossom ends off your cucumbers (b). These ends contain enzymes that can contribute to "hollow pickle syndrome" (see page 68).

3   Combine the chlorine-free water and salt in the pitcher, and add any starter or vinegar, if using.

4   Place the seasonings and tannin providers at the bottom of the jar or crock, followed by the cucumbers (c).

5   Pour the brine into the crock (d).

6   Weight everything down in such a way that it stays submerged (e).

7   If needed, cover the top of the jar or crock with the cloth, and affix the cloth with the rubber band.

8   Store at cool room temperature. Every day after the second or third, pull out a pickle, cut off a piece with a clean knife, and taste it. When the pickles are pleasantly sour but still crunchy, they are done. Move them to a cool place (like the refrigerator) immediately.

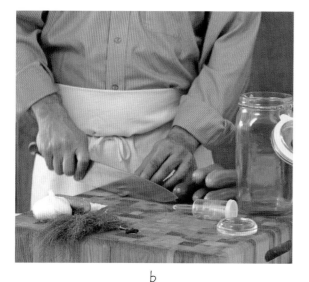

b

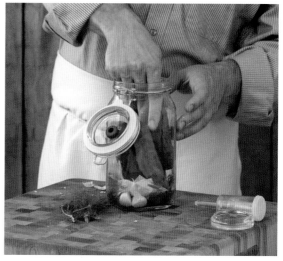

c

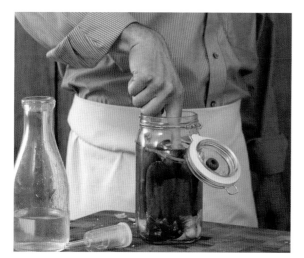

e

If a little mold grows on the top of the brine, it's not a problem—just remove it and carry on. But if there is a lot of mold, and it has long tendrils reaching down into the brine, it is a problem. Chalk one up to experience, send your pickles to the compost heap, and use more starter and/or vinegar next time.

See earlier in this chapter for pickle seasoning ideas and for suggestions about how to ensure the success of your pickles.

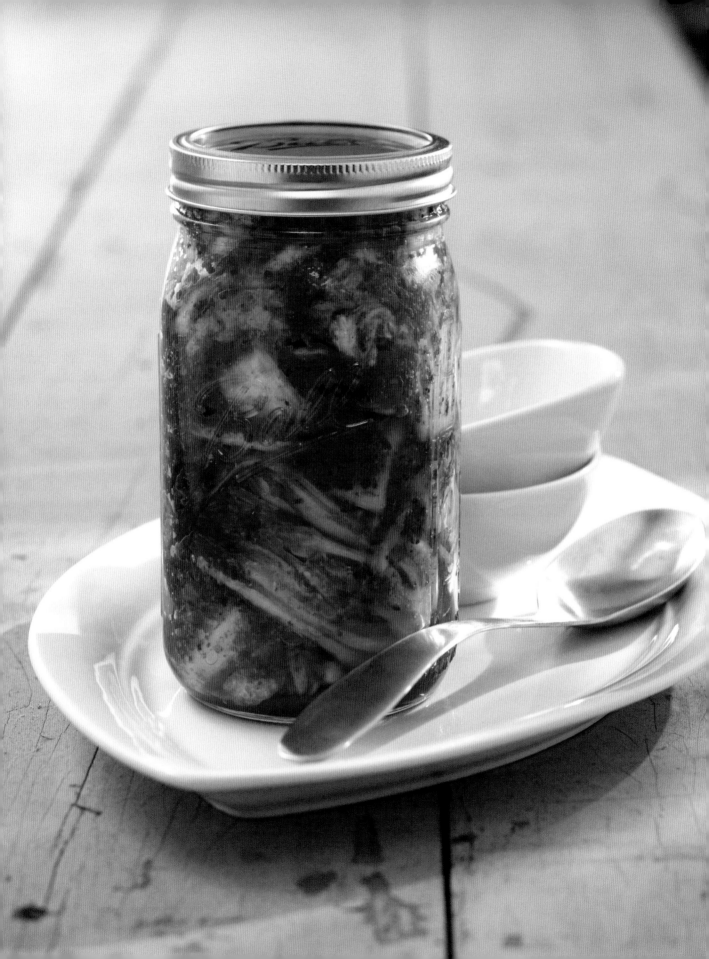

# KIMCHI

Kimchi (also *gimchi* and, especially in Hawaii, *kimchee* or *kim chee*) is a Korean fermented vegetable dish. Kimchi can showcase a variety of vegetables, but kimchi made from napa cabbage, also known as celery cabbage or Chinese cabbage, is the most iconic.

There's no one right or wrong way to spell "kimchi" in English (or to be more precise, in Roman characters). There is some amount of interpretation involved with transliterating words from one writing system into another, so it's possible to make a case for various spellings.

In my opinion, any fermented vegetable mix containing cruciferous vegetables (such as cabbage or radish), allium (such as garlic, onion, or scallion), ginger, and salt may safely be called kimchi. Other combinations of ingredients are also sometimes called kimchi.

Red pepper features prominently in many kimchis, but not in all of them. In fact, the first historical record of preserved cabbage in Asia predates the introduction of red pepper, a New World spice, by at least 2,000 years; so in relative terms, red pepper is a recent addition to kimchi.

Some might say that kimchi is a Korean sort of sauerkraut; others would say that sauerkraut is a European version of kimchi. In fact, the oldest known preserved cabbage was in China, so it may in fact be the Chinese who have the best claim to primacy!

*Recipe continued on page 89*

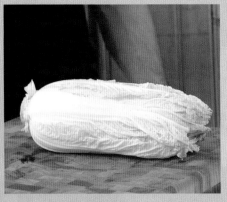

a

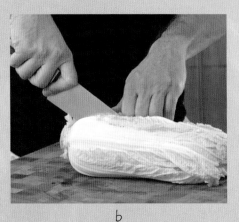

b

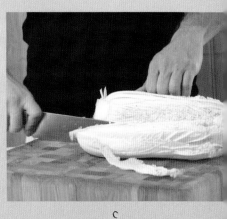

c

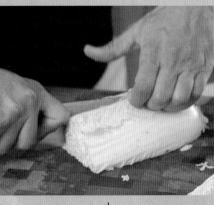

d

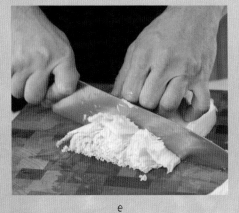

e

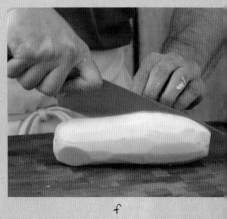

f

## CUTTING NAPA CABBAGE AND DAIKON

Napa cabbages (a) are typically more cylindrical than other varieties of cabbage, which are more spherical.

This makes napa cabbage easy to work with. Once you cut it in half the long way (b), (c), you can lay it down on your cutting board and quarter it (d), then start cutting it into even widths (e).

Daikon is equally convenient to handle. Rather than being small and round, it is large and cylindrical. So you can cut it lengthwise (f), and then easily slice it (g).

g

## INGREDIENTS

⅓ cup (100 g) coarse salt

2 cups (500 ml) nonchlorinated water

2 pounds (900 g) vegetables: napa cabbage, plus optional mustard greens, bok choy, or daikon

½ head garlic

1 large or 2 small onions

1 piece (½ inch, or 13 mm) gingerroot

Up to ½ cup (30 g) Korean red pepper powder, chopped or ground red peppers, or pepper flakes

1 tablespoon (15 g) sugar

1 teaspoon fish sauce (optional)

a few scallions or a length of Korean "long onion" (which is, more or less, a mature scallion)

## EQUIPMENT

Large mixing bowl

Large knife (a chef's knife is ideal)

Large cutting board (wood is ideal)

Vegetable peeler

Colander

Food processor (optional)

Wooden spoon

Wide-mouthed mason jars (2 pints [475 ml each], or 1 quart [950 ml])

*Recipe continued on page 90*

**Yield: Approximately 1 quart (950 ml), or 2 pounds (900 g)**

**Prep time: 10 minutes + overnight + 20 minutes**

**Total time: 5 days**

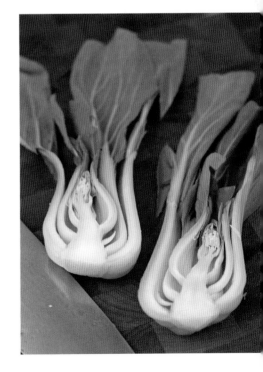

Kimchi continued

## PREPARATION

1   In the mixing bowl, dissolve the salt in the water to make a brine.

2   Cut up any or all of the 2 pounds (900 g) of vegetables: Quarter the leafy bunches of vegetables, or cut them into 1-inch (2.5 cm) square pieces. Slice the cabbage core and include as much or as little as you like. Peel the root vegetables, and cut them into thin diagonal slices, 1 inch (2.5 cm) or so long.

3   Put the cut vegetables into the brine and mix, using clean hands. The brine makes the vegetables more malleable. Cover the bowl to keep it free of foreign objects. After 6 or so hours (or overnight), drain the vegetables thoroughly in a colander. Taste them. They should be salty, but not unpleasantly so. If they are unpleasantly salty, rinse them or soak them in fresh nonchlorinated water, taste them again, and repeat until you are satisfied. Set them aside.

4   Peel the garlic and the onions. Peel the ginger (the edge of a spoon works nicely) (a).

5   Blend the onions, garlic, and ginger in a food processor (b), adding enough water to allow them to blend (c). (Or mix them with a mortar and pestle, or chop them finely with a knife.)

6   Add the red pepper (d), sugar, and fish sauce, if using, to the combination from step 5, adding just enough water to keep things blending into a paste.

7   Cut the scallions diagonally into 1-inch (2.5-cm) lengths (e), add them to the paste, and mix the paste with a wooden spoon.

8   Move the drained vegetables into a large bowl (f), and mix them with the seasoning paste using the spoon (g), (h). Taste the kimchi. If it is not salty enough, add more salt now and stir.

9   Pack the kimchi tightly into the Mason jars, leaving 1 inch (2.5 cm) of space at the top. Try to pack it down well enough to squeeze out most of the air bubbles along the side of the jar (i). Close the jar.

10  Leave the jar on the counter at room temperature for a few days. Taste it every day or two. It should start to taste a bit "wild." When you like the way it tastes, put it in a cool cellar or a refrigerator to store, or bury it in the ground. The cooler the temperature, the slower the subsequent fermentation.

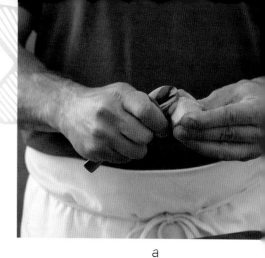

a

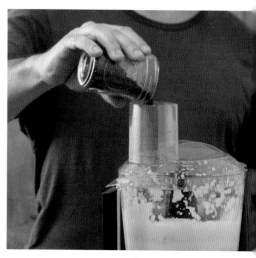

c

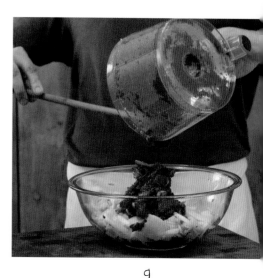

g

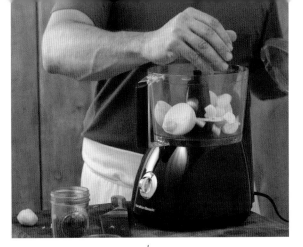

b

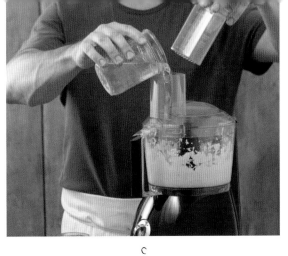

c

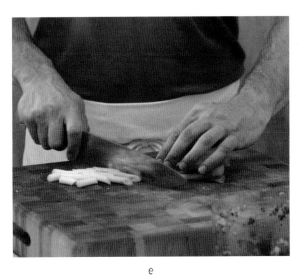

e

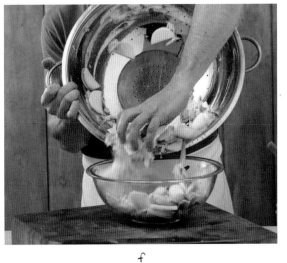

f

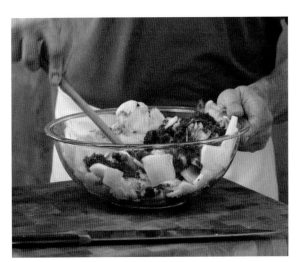

h

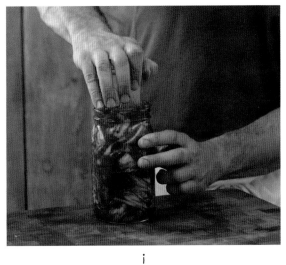

i

* You don't have to brine the vegetables first, but this is the traditional technique, and your kimchi may age better if you do.

* You can use other kinds of cabbage in place of napa—especially if you are in the midst of a national kimchi crisis (see below).

* Experiment with using less red pepper, or even none at all. The ginger flavor comes through more strongly when there is no red pepper.

* The vegetables can be cut however you like: 1-inch (2.5-cm) squares are just one possibility. For instance, you can shred everything to get a "slaw"-style kimchi. Conversely, you can leave the cabbages in quarters, or even just cut them part of the way through and stuff them with the spice mix. The more coarsely they are cut, the more important the brining is.

* You can try adding different things to your kimchi. Fruits and spices provide lots of possibilities: apples, Asian pears, citrus juice, curry powder, Chinese five-spice powder, and so on.

## THE KIMCHI CRISIS OF 2010

Kimchi is a staple food in Korea, eaten three times a day by many. And the most common variety of kimchi is made with napa cabbage. When heavy September rains compromised the South Korean cabbage crop in 2010, the price of a head of cabbage more than tripled, and it was a national crisis. The government had to take action; they implemented a kimchi relief plan, which included:

* rationing kimchi,

* paying subsidies to Korean cabbage farmers to reduce prices,

* lowering trade barriers that normally discouraged the import of cabbage from China, and even

* promoting the consumption of the less desirable "round" (green) cabbage.

## SERVING IDEAS FOR KIMCHI

* Fresh kimchi is great with grilled or smoked foods and goes especially nicely with pork and/or apples. So grilled pork chops, pulled pork, and grilled mackerel or seared tuna would go nicely with kimchi.

* Kimchi can take the place of plain sauerkraut in many contexts. For instance, if you use kimchi instead of sauerkraut, a Reuben sandwich becomes a Kimchi Reuben sandwich, adding a whole new dimension to the classic. (By the way, corned beef is fermented; see page 162.)

* Older, less crunchy kimchi can be used in cooked preparations like soups and stews, egg dishes, savory pancakes, and fried rice. *Kimchi jjigae* is a kimchi stew popular in Korea. Kimchi scrambled eggs might be just the thing on a cold winter morning.

* You can make a kimchi canapé with a cracker, an oatcake, or a toast square topped with Cheddar cheese, a slice of crispy apple, and a dollop of finely chopped kimchi. Raise some eyebrows at your next cocktail party!

* Grilled cheese with kimchi is another nice variation on a comfort food favorite.

* Top your baked potato with sour cream and kimchi. (Sour cream, as you might guess, is a fermented food, too; see page 107.)

* Try oysters on the half shell with kimchi juice. Who needs hot sauce and lemon?

* Kimchi nachos provide that south-of-the-thirty-eighth-parallel flavor.

* Kimchitini! Have a vodka cocktail with a hint of kimchi juice . . . or a big splash if you like it dirty.

* A kimchi Bloody Mary is perfect with brunch.

* For a Kimchi Michelada, combine a light-bodied beer, kimchi juice, and lime juice over ice in a salt-rimmed glass. It's cold and refreshing on a hot summer day.

# CHAPTER 5
# DAIRY

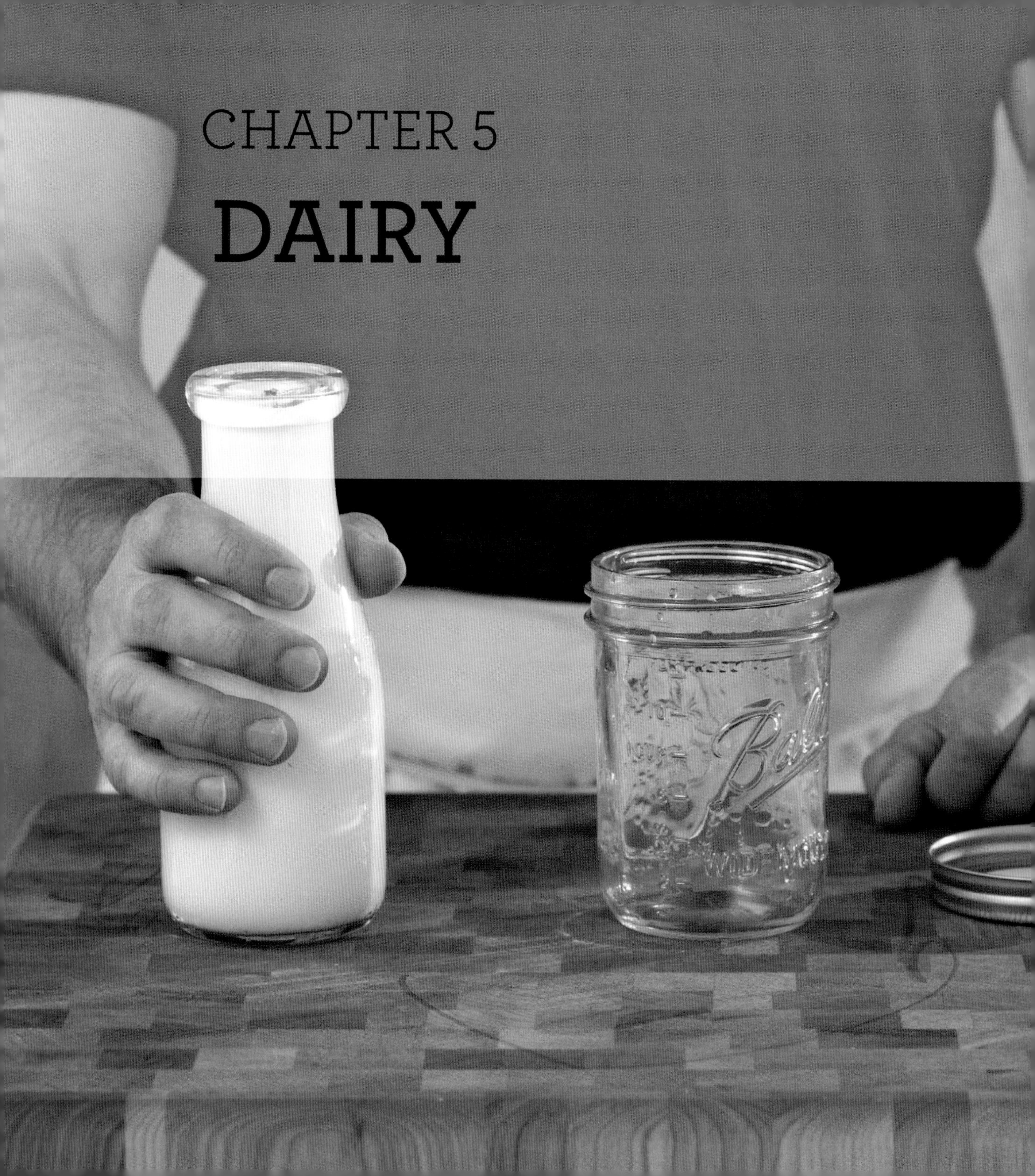

IN MANY PARTS OF THE WORLD, it's easy to go to the store, buy some milk, bring it home, and put it in the refrigerator, to be consumed over the course of the next week or so. The milk may have been drawn from animals hundreds or thousands of miles away, weeks before it was bought.

This has not always been possible.

A hundred years ago, homes did not have electrically powered refrigerators and freezers. Some homes had iceboxes: insulated boxes kept cool by large blocks of ice. Iceboxes were neither universal nor convenient, and ice was expensive and perishable.

So in the past, storage of milk was an issue. After several hours at typical room temperatures, fresh milk was no longer fresh, so it was necessary to find ways to extend its life. There are various excellent options, and many of them involve fermentation.

# WHICH MILK SHOULD I BUY?

When making fermented milk products, the better and healthier the milk you start with, the better your results will be. Raw, unpasteurized milk is the best because it has been processed the least. It is relatively easy to get in some parts of the world, and difficult to get and/or illegal in others. If raw milk is not an option for you, try to find pasteurized milk that is not homogenized. If you have a choice between pasteurized and ultrapasteurized, get pasteurized. Beyond that, whole milk is better than reduced-fat milk.

Milk from cows that have grazed on grass is preferable to milk from cows that have been fed grain, for a variety of reasons. It will contain more of vitamins A, D, E, and $K_2$. Also, cows are not well suited to grain-heavy diets, so grain-fed cattle tend to get more infections, which leads to increased antibiotic use. Although milk from cows with active infections is generally discarded, the whole cycle of feeding cattle grain and antibiotics is best avoided.

If you are in a country like the United States that allows genetically modified artificial growth hormones (rBST or rBGH) to be injected into dairy animals, consider buying milk from producers who do not follow this practice. Raw milk and milk from smaller farms are often free of these hormones; organic milk is always free of them; and even some nonorganic large-scale milk distributors label their milk as being "rBST-free" or "rBGH-free."

## MILK FROM OTHER ANIMALS

Milk from cows and buffalo is the most popular milk in much of the world, and the easiest to get. But humans consume the milk of many other animals besides bovines. You may have access to milk from goats, sheep, camels, horses, zebras, or any other mammals. Each is different. Recipes in this book are written with cow's milk in mind. If you use milk from other animals, you might need to adjust fermenting times, because of the different compositions of these milks.

## NONDAIRY "MILKS"

Recently, nondairy beverages marketed as "milks" have appeared on store shelves: soy milk, rice milk, almond milk, and hemp milk, for example. They can generally be made by grinding and boiling their ingredients in water and then straining off the resulting liquid. In practice, however, industrial food manufacturers use hexane and other toxic solvents to accelerate the process; they do additional processing and add sweeteners and flavorings to create a more saleable product. These "milks" are often marketed as healthy alternatives to dairy milk, especially for vegans and for people who have trouble drinking pasteurized cow milk.

Unfortunately, many of these industrially produced and sweetened nondairy alternatives are not healthy. Soy milk is particularly problematic because:

* toxic solvents are often used in its manufacture;

* it undergoes intensive processing to neutralize its bitter taste;

* more than 90 percent of the soybeans grown in the United States are genetically modified; and

* when consumed in large amounts, soy is a potent endocrine disruptor.

And many alternative milks, not just soy, can contain sugar and other sweeteners that have been added to make them more palatable. Sometimes they contain colorings to make them whiter as well.

So if you are thinking of buying alternative milks for health reasons, please do your research, and definitely read labels. If there is anything in the ingredients list that you don't understand, you may not want to buy it. And watch out for sweeteners, GMOs, and large amounts of soy.

Having said all of this, nondairy milks can often successfully be made into yogurt and kefir. Nondairy yogurts can even be found in stores and can be used as starters. Results may vary from one nondairy milk to another, even from brand to brand, so it is hard to say anything categorical about how dairy recipes should be changed to accommodate nondairy ingredients; be prepared to adjust recipes and improvise as needed.

## LACTOSE INTOLERANCE

Some children and many adults have trouble digesting lactose, a carbohydrate occurring naturally in dairy milk. For them, drinking fresh milk and consuming some milk products can result in bloating, gas, and discomfort. This is generally because their bodies are not able to generate enough lactase, the enzyme that breaks down lactose. Instead, the lactose ferments in their intestines and causes gas.

Dairy products that are fermented can be much easier to digest because they contain smaller amounts of lactose. Microbes have already digested some or most of the original lactose in the milk. Much of this lactose gets converted into lactic acid, which is what gives fermented milk products their characteristic sour flavor.

Also note that raw milk contains the lactase enzyme. So many who are "lactose intolerant" and have trouble with pasteurized milk have no problem at all with raw milk. In fact, consuming raw milk can help you digest other milk products that might have given you problems otherwise (like ice cream!).

While raw milk contains the lactase enzyme, pasteurized milk does not because pasteurization destroys it, along with other enzymes and heat-sensitive vitamins. To compensate for this loss, pasteurized milk is often fortified with synthetic vitamins. These vitamins may be harder for the body to absorb than their natural counterparts.

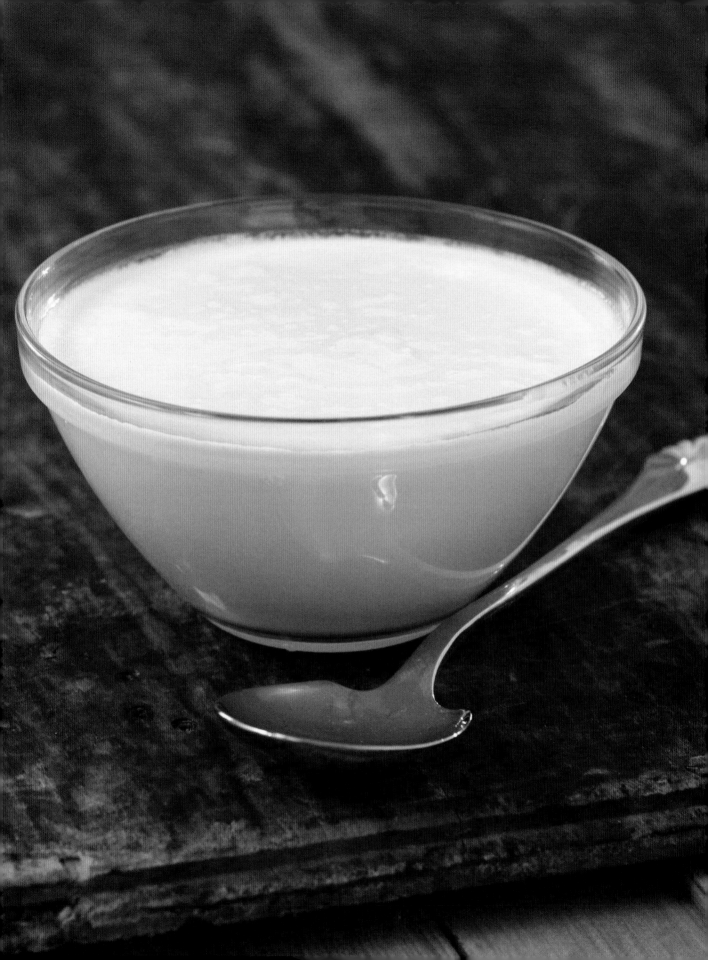

# YOGURT

It is likely that yogurt originated accidentally in the Middle East more than 4,500 years ago. Options for transporting milk (and other liquids) were limited; putting the milk in animal skins was a good option because the skins were available and water-proof. A plausible scenario: The natural bacteria from an animal skin could have combined with milk, and along with the warm temperatures, could have led to something we would recognize today as yogurt. Once the yogurt culture had found a home in this animal skin, the same skin could be used to make a new batch, or the yogurt itself could be used as a starter.

People have eaten yogurt for millennia; it is a traditional food around the Mediterra-nean and in western, central, and southern Asia. In recent years, it has found its way to North America, northern Europe, and even to parts of the Far East, where it is one of the few dairy products consumed.

Yogurt is produced by bacterial fermentation of milk at warm temperatures. The precise collection of bacteria varies somewhat from one sample to another, and different bacteria result in different tastes and textures. It is typically made by heating milk, rendering it more or less sterile; allowing the milk to cool to around 110°F (43°C); then introducing the desired collection of bacteria to the milk and keeping it warm for long enough to allow the bacteria to do their work.

## INGREDIENTS

6 tablespoons (90 g) yogurt, as a starter (see page 101)

1 quart (950 ml) milk, less 6 tablespoons (90 g)

## EQUPMENT

1-quart (950 ml) or two 1-pint (475-ml) mason jar(s)

Medium saucepan

Food thermometer

Incubator big enough to hold all your mason jars (an insulated bag or cooler, a pilot light–style oven that can stay at approximately 110°F [45°C], a food dehydrator with the thermostat set at 110°F [45°C], or a yogurt maker!)

A few extra mason jars of any size

**Yield: 1 quart (950 ml)**

**Prep time: 10 minutes**

**Total time: 12–24 hours**

*Recipe continued on page 100*

## PREPARATION

1 Measure out the yogurt that you're going to use as a starter (a). Put it in the quart jar, or split it equally between the pint jars.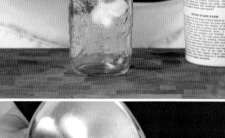

2 Heat the milk in the saucepan until it is almost 180°F (80°C). Take it off the heat and let it cool to 110°F (45°C), or a little warmer. If you are impatient, you may set your pan in cold water or an ice bath, and/or pour the milk into a metal mixing bowl to allow it to cool more quickly.

3 Add the milk to the jar, leaving 1 inch (2.5 cm) or so of room at the top (b). Close the jar and shake it so that the yogurt starter mixes well with the milk (c).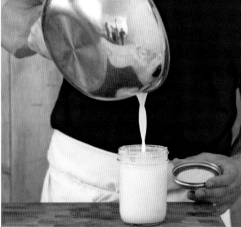

4 Put the jar(s) in the warm or insulated incubator you have prepared (d). If your incubator does not have a heat source of its own, fill some of your extra mason jars with hot tap water (130°F–140°F [55°C–60°C]) and put them in the incubator alongside your yogurt jar(s).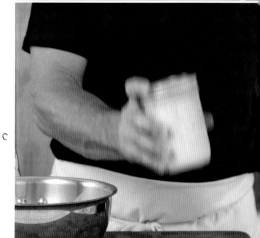

5 After 12 to 24 hours, your yogurt will be ready. If you like, put it in the refrigerator, where it will thicken further.

Yogurt will keep in the refrigerator for at least two weeks, and probably longer. After a week or two, it may start to separate, and clear liquid may rise to the top; this is not a problem, and it doesn't mean that the yogurt is spoiling. The clear liquid is yogurt whey, which is explained in the next recipe.

## SOME SERVING IDEAS FOR YOUR HOMEMADE YOGURT

Yogurt can be served in a variety of ways. Of course it can be eaten plain, on its own. You can also serve it with a little honey or maple syrup, with some berries or fruit, or even with some fermented fruit chutney (see page 120) for a double dose of fermented foods! It can also be mixed with chopped vegetables, herbs, and other seasonings. Beyond that, yogurt can be used as the base for smoothies, milkshakes, or soups, and it can be used in any recipe that calls for milk or sour cream. It also frequently accompanies savory Middle Eastern and Indian dishes.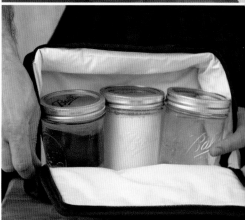

a

b

c

d

## YOGURT STARTERS

The better the starter, the better the resulting yogurt. Typically, a portion of an existing batch of yogurt is used as a starter to get the desired bacteria into a new batch. Use homemade yogurt as a starter if you have some. Otherwise, buy the best yogurt you can from the store. Find yogurt that is minimally processed. It should be plain, whole-milk yogurt and as fresh as possible; it should not contain any funny stuff like gelatin or nonfat dry milk powder; and it must contain active yogurt cultures. Read the label carefully. Also, use younger yogurt rather than older. The longer yogurt sits the less active its bacteria will be because once they have finished "eating" the lactose in the yogurt, they have nothing more to eat, and they gradually die off.

**Important note:** If, and only if, you are starting with raw milk, you may skip the sterilization stage and simply bring the milk up to the favorable temperature range, add your starter, and maintain the temperature. Yogurt made this way will contain a greater variety of beneficial microbes, which is good from a health point of view; however the results will be less predictable, and the yogurt may be thinner than yogurt made from heated milk, so its texture will be less predictable.

## CHEESE

Making milk into cheese is yet another way of preserving it, as well as making it easier to transport. Cheese is made by coagulating some of the milk proteins and removing most of the liquid. This liquid is called whey, or cheese whey. Cheese whey is different from yogurt whey (see page 102) because cheesemaking often involves heating the milk, in which case the whey does not contain live bacteria and is therefore not usable as a starter.

Cheeses go through a curding, or curdling, process. Milk is acidulated either by adding an acid, such as lemon juice or vinegar, or by fermenting with specific bacteria. Sometimes it is heated. Whey may be drained off. If you are making curd cheeses such as ricotta, farmers' cheese, Quark, or paneer, you may be done at this point. These cheeses are not much more complicated than curdled milk.

Otherwise, we continue the curdling process with the addition of enzymes, either rennet derived from animal sources or alternative enzymes from plants or fungi. For different results, we use different amounts of enzymes, different ultimate moisture levels, different types of bacteria, more or less salt, more or less aging, sometimes a particular mold, sometimes a coating of wax, and sometimes other sorts of treatments.

This book does not include recipes for cheesemaking, which it is its own entire field of knowledge. It is easy to find articles, books, and even schools dedicated to cheesemaking. See Resources on page 168 for some top recommended reading.

 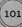

# STRAINED YOGURT AND WHEY

When yogurt is left to strain through cheesecloth or muslin, the results are thick, strained yogurt (also known as Greek-style yogurt or *labneh*) and thin yogurt whey, which is the liquid that drains off. Strained yogurt is thicker and richer than regular yogurt and is less inclined to curdle, which makes it usable in some culinary contexts where regular yogurt might not be. Strained yogurt is a delicious spread on bread, for instance, and works nicely to enrich sauces. It is also often served with fruit or honey as a dessert or breakfast.

Yogurt whey is useful in fermenting vegetables and fruits because it is an excellent source of the right sorts of bacteria. (For more instructions on fermenting with whey, see page 72.) It is also a great probiotic drink, pleasantly sour and easy to digest.

## INGREDIENTS

1 quart (900 g) plain yogurt (homemade or store-bought)

## EQUIPMENT

Fine cheesecloth (if possible, find cheesecloth that is not bleached with chlorine)

Large fine-mesh strainer

Mixing bowl or pitcher to suspend the strainer over

Wooden spoon (optional)

**Yield: Approximately 1 pint (450 g) strained yogurt and 1 pint (475 ml) whey**

**Prep time: 5–20 minutes**

**Total time: 4–12 hours**

## PREPARATION

1 Moisten the cheesecloth with chlorine-free tap water, and lay it on the inside of the strainer. (By moistening the cheesecloth ahead of time, you minimize the amount of whey that the cheesecloth absorbs.)

2 Put the strainer over the bowl or pitcher.

3 Scoop, spoon, or pour the yogurt into the strainer (a), and let it drain (b).

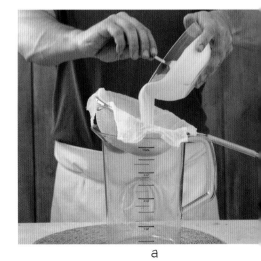

a

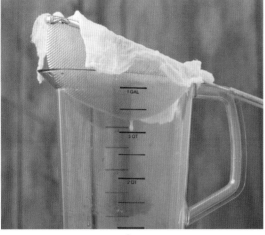

b

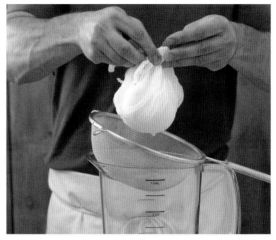

c

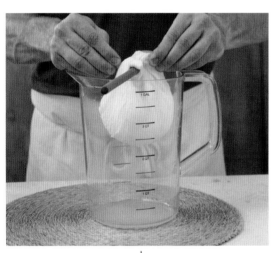

d

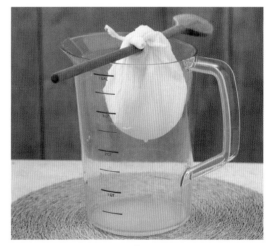

e

4 When the yogurt has drained a bit, you may, if you wish, try to tie the ends of the cheesecloth around the handle of the spoon in such a way that it can continue to drain into the bowl or pitcher (c), (d), (e). If you don't do this, then cover the strainer with a plate or something similar to keep foreign objects out of the yogurt.

5 When the yogurt has thickened, put it in a sealed container and refrigerate it; it will continue to thicken as it cools in the refrigerator. Put the whey in the refrigerator, too. Consume them both within a couple of weeks, although they may last longer. When they have started to go bad, you will know because they will get slimy or moldy.

# KEFIR

Kefir is a fermented milk food that is a close relative to yogurt, though generally thinner in consistency. The origin of kefir is a matter of some speculation. Some accounts hold that it has existed in central Asia since at least 3000 BCE; a legend tells that it was a gift from Allah to Muhammad.

Regardless, the starters necessary to make kefir were guarded by the people of the region until the early twentieth century, at which time a Russian spy supposedly stole some of the starters and brought them to Moscow, whence they spread far and wide. Today, kefir is enjoyed in some of the same places yogurt is. Because of its generally thinner consistency, it is more likely to be consumed as a drink or as a component in a drink, in place of milk, or in a soup. The biggest practical differences between kefir and yogurt are (1) the microbes responsible for kefir are industrious at room temperature, while yogurt's are most productive above about 100°F (40°C); and (2) a kefir starter is a cottage cheese–like collection of globules, referred to as "grains," which is strained out and reused repeatedly.

Kefir grains are combinations of yeasts and bacteria living on a substrate made up of a variety of dairy components. After you use them to start your batch of kefir, you can strain them out and save them to start your next batch. Each time you use them, they grow slightly in size. You can get kefir starters at health food stores, via the Internet, or if you're very lucky, from a friend.

## INGREDIENTS

1 quart (950 ml) milk, or a little less

1–2 tablespoons (15-30 g) kefir grains

Yield: 1 quart (950 ml)

Prep time: 5–20 minutes

Total time: 12–24 hours

## EQUIPMENT

Medium saucepan (optional)

Food thermometer (optional)

Two 1-quart (950 ml) mason jars

Small strainer, ideally sized to the mouth of the mason jar

Mixing bowl or pitcher to suspend the strainer over

Wooden spoon (optional)

## PREPARATION

1  If you like, you may heat the milk in a saucepan to 180°F (80°C), and allow it to cool to below 100°F (40°C). Doing this ensures that there are no other microbes living in the milk. This step is not really necessary because the microbes from the kefir will probably come pretty quickly to dominate any other microbes present in the milk.

2  Fill one jar most of the way with milk, leaving some space at the top (1 inch, or 2.5 cm, is sufficient), and then add the kefir grains (a).

3  Put the lid on the jar and shake it (b).

4  Keep the jar at room temperature for 12 to 24 hours (a little less if your room is warm, perhaps a little more if it's cold). Shake it every few hours, if you think of it.

5  Shake the jar one last time. Set the strainer over the second mason jar, and strain the kefir into it (c), (d). Straining allows you to recover your kefir grains (starter).

6  Put a lid on the jar and store the finished kefir in the refrigerator, where it might keep for months, or on the counter, where it might keep for weeks. At some point, it will start to separate, and eventually, it will get unpleasantly sour and yeasty; it will become unappetizing before it becomes unsafe to eat.

7  You may use your kefir grains to start another batch of kefir immediately. Otherwise, rinse them in nonchlorinated water, then store them in a small jar of nonchlorinated water in the refrigerator until the next time you want to use them.

The trickiest part of the kefir-making process is the straining. Especially if you are using unhomogenized milk, it can be difficult to distinguish grains of the kefir starter from bits of milk fat. Shaking the kefir is good because it will break up the milk fat but not the kefir grains. Also, the sooner you strain the kefir, the less clumpy it will be, and the easier to strain. In any case, it need not be a precise process; nothing bad will happen if, on the one hand, you strain out some of the fat and save it with the starter or, on the other hand, you eat some of the kefir grains. (Just don't eat them all, or you won't be able to make another batch!)

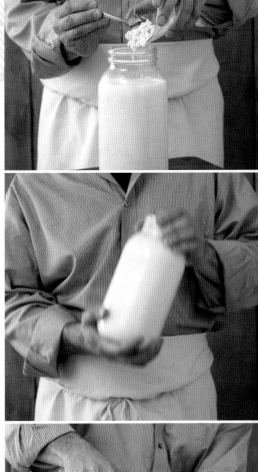

a

b

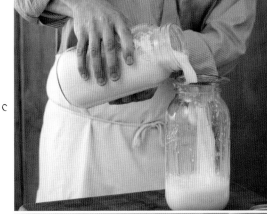

c

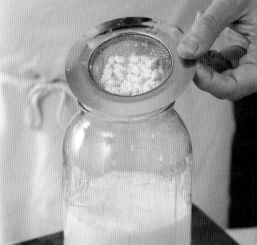

d

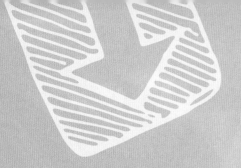

## MAKING FLAVORED YOGURT AND KEFIR

In the store we encounter a dizzying array of yogurt products, and, increasingly, a variety of kefirs as well. How do we choose among them? When at the store, I encourage careful label reading. Yogurt and kefir should contain milk (ideally whole milk) and starter culture. They might contain some fruit, or perhaps a natural sweetener like honey or maple syrup. Anything beyond that probably spells trouble. For instance, many "lite" yogurts may contain gelatin, cornstarch, nonfat milk powder, and artificial sweeteners. None of these belong in yogurt or kefir.

This array of questionable yogurt products and kefir in the store is further encouragement for us to make our own, where we can see and control exactly what is going into it.

Once you've mastered making your own and you would like to have flavored yogurt and kefir at home, your best bet is to make it plain and then add fresh fruit, preserved fruit, or sweetener when you are about to eat it. You can also add things that aren't sweet, like cucumbers, garlic, dill, fennel, caraway, mint, and so on.

## YOGURT VERSUS KEFIR

Yogurt and kefir are similar and have many of the same virtues. They are both preserved, fermented, soured milk products. They are both very popular in various parts of the world, in savory and sweet preparations, or on their own. They both have nutritive and digestive benefits for those who eat them because of their live cultures. You may have personal preferences that lead you to make and eat one more than the other. You may also have a particular favorite recipe that calls specifically for either yogurt or kefir, or one that is best made with either a thicker or a thinner sour dairy product.

Aside from thickness, they're more or less interchangeable in recipes. All else being equal, I favor kefir over yogurt, for a few reasons:

★ It's easier to maintain the temperature required to make kefir (room temperature) than it is to maintain the temperature required to make yogurt (above body temperature)—unless, of course, you live in a very hot climate! Perhaps because of this, I find that my kefir always turns out well, but my yogurt sometimes fails: It can separate immediately, fail to thicken, or acquire a funny smell.

★ Yogurt gives the most consistent good results when you heat and cool the milk before adding the starter to it; kefir can work well whether or not you heat and cool the milk. The heating and cooling take some time and effort. Also, especially if you are using raw milk, heat will destroy some of the vitamins and enzymes in the milk.

★ Kefir generally contains a wider range of microbes, including bacteria and yeast, than yogurt does. This is even more true if the kefir has been made from unheated raw milk, in which case it may also have more natural vitamins. So, very loosely speaking, kefir's potential health benefits may be greater than yogurt's.

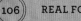

# CRÈME FRAÎCHE

*Crème fraîche* literally means "fresh cream" in French; despite this, crème fraîche is the name given to cream that has been soured.

Originally, crème fraîche was simply unpasteurized cream that had been left out and allowed to ferment through the action of lactic acid bacteria. This same method does not work with pasteurized cream because the lactic acid bacteria are destroyed in the pasteurization process. For those who cannot get unpasteurized cream, an alternative is to start with pasteurized cream, warm the cream, add a starter culture, and let it ferment. Options for starter cultures include yogurt, kefir, and cultured buttermilk (which is available at most supermarkets) (see page 111 for a discussion of buttermilk). Using buttermilk probably gets you closest to what unpasteurized cream would do on its own. Or, if you have a previous batch of homemade crème fraîche, that is an excellent starter!

Crème fraîche typically has a butterfat content of 30 to 40 percent. What is called sour cream in the United States is similar to crème fraîche but is made from a mixture of cream and milk (half-and-half) and typically weighs in at about 18 percent to 20 percent butterfat. The sour cream you buy at the store all too frequently contains thickening and acidifying agents, and sometimes flavorings of various sorts. You can also buy "lite" sour cream, which has less fat and more additives, and even nonfat sour cream, which has no fat and still more additives. Store-bought sour cream, like store-bought crème fraîche, has often been pasteurized after fermentation, so it can't be used as a starter. If you have bought some sour cream or crème fraîche from the store and you're not sure about it, don't use it as a starter; it's easier to use buttermilk or yogurt.

Making sour cream at home is a bit harder than making crème fraîche, and the result is a bit less luxurious, so why not make crème fraîche? But if you would like to make sour cream, it's best to try to regulate its temperature as you would when making yogurt.

*Recipe continued on page 109*

## STORE-BOUGHT CRÈME FRAÎCHE

Be aware that store-bought crème fraîche has often been pasteurized after fermentation, so its bacteria have been killed. It is not useful as a starter, and it has lost its probiotic benefits. If it doesn't say "live cultures" on the packaging, then it's likely that it has been pasteurized after fermentation.

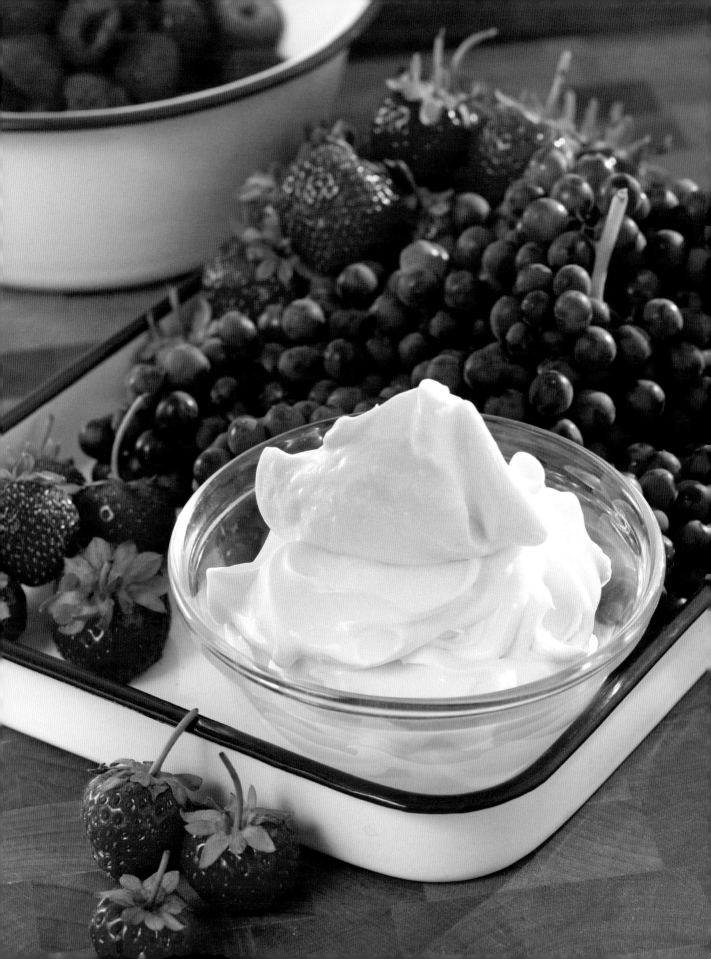

**Crème Fraîche continued**

You can make crème fraîche pretty much the way you make yogurt (see page 99), except that you can use different starters, and it is not as picky about temperature. It's possible to make it in a warm room without using any insulated or heated containers. If you can't get unpasteurized cream, pasteurized cream will do, with a starter. Ultra-pasteurized cream may not work well, even with a starter.

## INGREDIENTS

12–13 ounces (350–400 ml) unpasteurized cream

3 tablespoons (45 g) yogurt, kefir, or cultured buttermilk as a starter, if using pasteurized cream; starter is optional if using raw cream

**Yield: 1 pint (450 g)**

**Prep time: 10 minutes**

**Total time: 12–18 hours**

## EQUIPMENT

1-pint (475-ml) mason jar

## PREPARATION

1  If using a starter, measure out the amount you're going to use. Put it in the mason jar.

2  Add the cream to the jar, leaving 1 inch (2.5 cm) or so of room at the top. Close the jar and shake it so that the starter mixes well with the cream.

3  Place the jar somewhere warm for 12 hours or overnight. Check the cream. If it has not yet thickened, leave it for another 6 hours.

4  When it has thickened, store it in the refrigerator, where it will keep for a week or two.

Crème fraîche is great for cooking because it won't curdle the way cream sometimes does when you heat it or add an acid like lemon juice or vinegar.

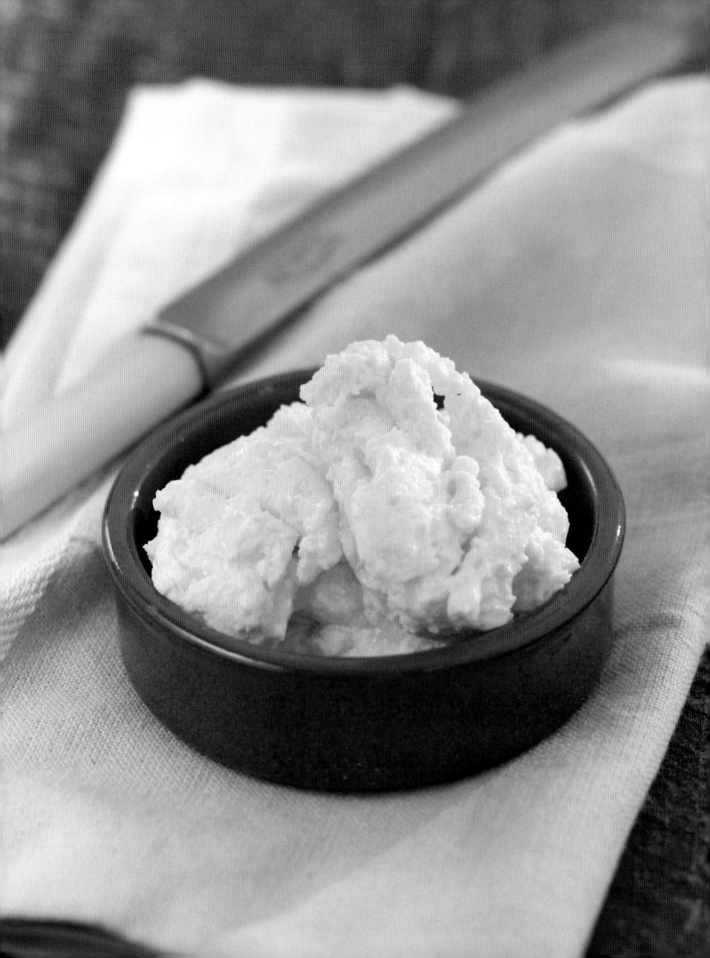

# BUTTER AND BUTTERMILK

Making cream into crème fraîche is one way to preserve it. By making it more acidic, you are making it less prone to spoilage. Another way to preserve cream is to turn it into butter, thus removing most of the water and carbohydrates from it, leaving a little protein and a lot of fat. In fact, you can get the best of both worlds by making crème fraîche and then turning it into butter!

When you make butter from pasteurized cream, you get what is called sweet cream butter. When you make it from fermented cream (like crème fraîche), using the same process, you get cultured butter.

In the old days, most butter was cultured butter, simply because cream was raw, refrigeration was difficult, and most cream had started to ferment on its own by the time folks had gathered enough of it to start making butter. Nowadays, we make cultured butter because it has a nicer flavor, it has healthy bacteria, and it keeps better. In fact, a lot of store-bought sweet cream butter has flavorings added to it to make it taste more like cultured butter. (Read the label and you'll see.)

If this is the case, then why doesn't everyone simply make cultured butter? Because cultured butter takes longer to make. If you are a small producer making it at home, the extra time isn't a big deal because you're going through the work of making the butter anyway. But if you are a large industrial producer, then time is money; using additives is cheaper, quicker, and more predictable than fermenting your cream.

Making butter is simple: you put cream in a jar, and shake the jar until the cream turns into butter. It's even easier if you have children: hand the jar over to them! You can also use a blender, mixer, or food processor if you have one.

When you are done, you will have butter, and you will have some residual liquid. This residual liquid is true buttermilk. The buttermilk you get from making cultured butter is more interesting than the buttermilk you get from making sweet cream butter: it has more flavor, is more acidic, and contains live cultures. Either way, genuine buttermilk is fat free, or pretty close to it, because the fat is in the butter.

The buttermilk you buy at the store is usually skim milk that has been fermented with a starter. It is quite similar to the buttermilk you get when you make cultured butter except that the store-bought buttermilk contains all of the milk proteins, whereas many of these proteins wind up in the butter and not in the concomitant buttermilk made at home. Cultured buttermilk, like cultured whey, can be used as a starter for other fermentation products. It is also a popular ingredient in recipes because of its flavor and its acidity, and microbes are useful in marinades because they can help tenderize meats.

*Recipe continued on page 112*

**Butter and Buttermilk continued**

**Yield: Varies**

**Prep time: 10–15 minutes**

**Total time: 10–15 minutes**

## INGREDIENTS

Cream or cultured cream (crème fraîche, for example)

Ice water

Sea salt (optional)

## EQUIPMENT

A couple of mason jars

Blender, food processor, stand mixer, or hand-held electric mixer (optional)

Small bowl

Medium bowl

Wooden spoon

Cutting board (with a channel, if available) (optional)

## PREPARATION

1  Put the cream in a mason jar (a), close the lid tightly, and shake it until it becomes solid (b). Alternatively, use your equipment to blend it until it solidifies (c).

2  Pour off the liquid into a small bowl (d).

3  Add some ice or ice water to your butter (e), and agitate it again (f). This will help draw off more liquid.

4  Using a wooden spoon or other instrument of your choice, transfer the butter to a meduim bowl or turn it out onto a cutting board.

5  Massage the butter with the wooden spoon to remove even more residual liquid (g). The more liquid you can remove, the better your butter will keep.

6  Before you're done massaging it, add salt to taste, if desired.

7  Refrigerate your butter. Optionally, once it has chilled and firmed up, massage it again to get more of the liquid out.

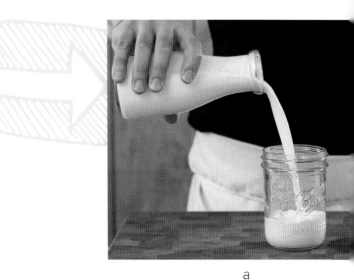

a

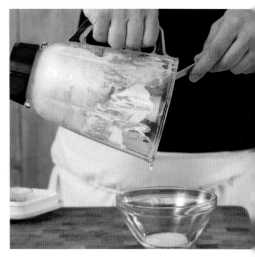

d

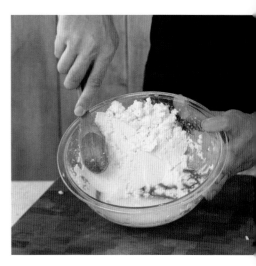

g

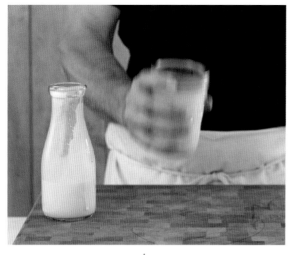

b

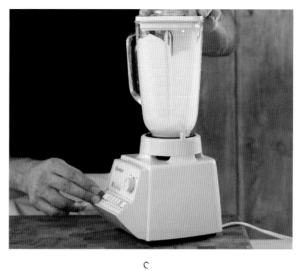

c

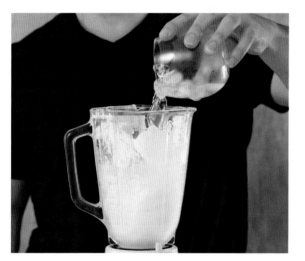

e

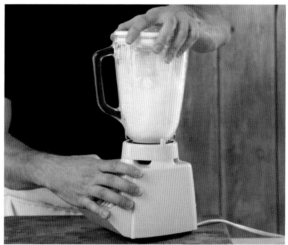

f

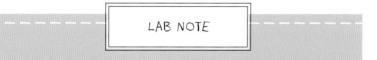

## LAB NOTE

If you decide to make cultured butter, you can use partially fermented cream. So, for instance, you can follow the procedure for making crème fraîche (page 107), but you don't have to let it ferment for quite as long.

# CHAPTER 6

# FERMENTED FRUIT CONDIMENTS

FRUIT, ESPECIALLY SOFT FRUIT, has a short shelf life at room temperature. Even in the refrigerator, it loses its appeal pretty quickly.

And when we grow it, soft fruit has the infuriating habit of becoming ripe all at once. By the end of summer, we may become blasé about perfectly ripe peaches, but come February, we may crave them. And the peaches in the supermarket will probably not be as good as the ones we found at the farmers' market in the summer.

FERMENTING FRUIT ALLOWS us to preserve the summer's bounty until a time when we can appreciate it again. Fermentation also allows us to develop sweet-and-sour flavors that might be better accompaniments for savory dishes, say, than the unrelenting delicious sweetness of fresh fruit.

Many soured foods we eat today can trace their roots to traditional bacterially fermented foods. We have seen that this is the case for vegetables and for dairy; it is also the case for fruit.

Sour fruit condiments can be wonderful accompaniments for flavorful meat, fish, grain, and vegetable dishes. Indian food, in some parts of India and in many parts of the world, is accompanied by mango chutneys, lime pickles, and all sorts of sour things. It's not hard to imagine fruit fermenting quickly in many of the hot climates of India. The sweet sourness of fermented fruit offsets the creaminess of butter-based dishes and helps cut through the dense textures of grain-based dishes.

Fermented fruit condiments are also good accompaniments for desserts such as dairy and pastries. Or fermented fruits can stand on their own as desserts. And some fermented fruits are great in a glass of sparkling water, with an added touch of sweetness perhaps.

Fermenting fruit can be trickier than fermenting vegetables. The high sugar content of many types of fruit tends to attract yeast, so if you are not assertive in guiding the fermentation, by using a bacterial starter, you may wind up with a fruit wine rather than a condiment. There is of course nothing wrong with fermenting fruit to get alcohol. However, alcohol is not the subject of this chapter—it is discussed in the next one!

Bacterial starters appropriate for fruit ferments are the same as those for vegetable ferments: whey, liquid from a previous ferment, or starter from an envelope.

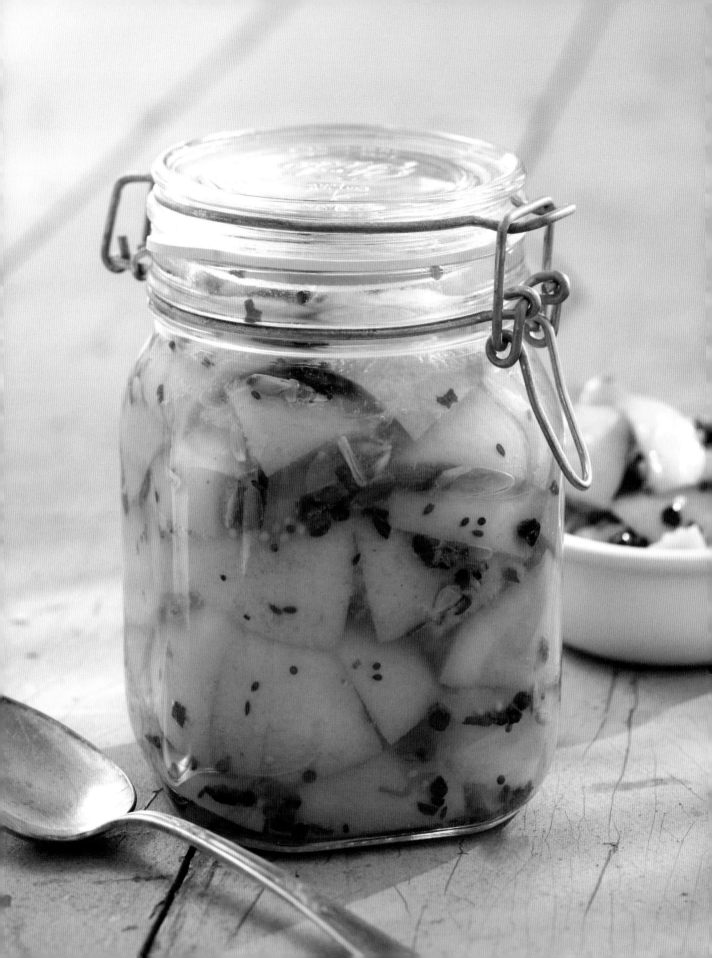

# PRESERVED LEMONS AND LIMES

When preserved, especially when preserved with spices, lemons and limes take on a complex, deep set of flavors. In addition, they can keep for months or even a year or longer, tasting more and more interesting as time goes on.

Preserved lemons are important in North African cooking. Limes preserved in the same way play a role in Southeast Asian cuisine. Either, or a mixture of both, can add a unique flavor to ceviche or cocktails. And in fact, squeezing a wedge or two of preserved citrus into a glass with some ice and a little sugar gives you a fantastic summer drink—Nature's own sports drink, with electrolytes and quick carbohydrates but none of the preservatives or colorings of commercial sports drinks: the ultimate lemonade.

Nonorganic citrus fruit accumulate pesticides in their rinds, so here it is very important to use organic lemons and limes . . . or lemons and limes from your own trees if you are lucky enough to have them.

## INGREDIENTS

1½ pounds (675 g) lemons and/or limes (about 5 or 6 lemons or 8 to 10 limes, depending on size), at room temperature

¼ cup (60 g) sea salt (see page 48)

Assorted spices of your choice: a cinnamon stick, a bay leaf, a few cloves, a few peppercorns, a handful of coriander seeds, or a shake of "pickling spice" (optional)

1 or 2 additional lemons, for juice

## EQUIPMENT

Large cutting board (wood is ideal)

A large knife (a chef's knife is ideal)

1-pint (475-ml) mason jar with a tight-fitting lid

**Yield: 1 pint (475 ml)**

**Prep time: 10 minutes**

**Total time: 6 months**

*Recipe continued on page 118*

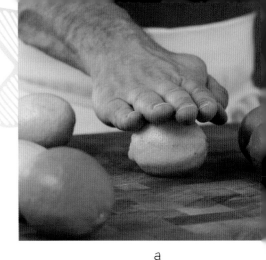

a

## PREPARATION

1 Take the lemons and/or limes out of the refrigerator an hour ahead of time to bring them to room temperature.

2 If they are waxed, or if you're not sure, blanch them in boiling water for 30 seconds, then take them out and let them cool.

3 Soften the fruit by rolling them on the counter under your palm, exerting some pressure, but not so much that the rinds split (a), (b).

4 Cut each lemon or lime along its equator (c). Then cut each hemisphere into four wedges (d); alternatively, make these cuts three-quarters of the way through but not all the way. Discard the seeds.

5 Put some salt in the bottom of the jar (e), add some spices, if using, and add a fruit's worth of wedges. Pack down firmly (f). Repeat this, layer by layer, until everything is in the jar, or the jar is nearly full (g). If the released juice does not cover the fruit, juice 1 or 2 additional fruit and add their juice to the jar. Close the jar, leaving 1 inch (2.5 cm) of headroom at the top.

6 Store the jar at room temperature, out of direct sunlight. For the first week, open the jar every day and pack it down so that the liquid rises to cover. The fruit start to change character after a week or two. Left at room temperature, they will continue to deepen in flavor for a year or so. Put them in the refrigerator at any time to slow their progress.

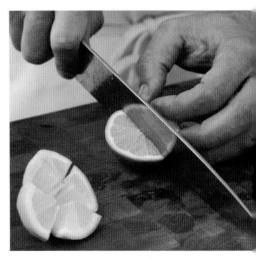

d

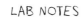

### LAB NOTES

A little white mold may grow on the top of the lemons or limes, especially if the juice is low. This is not a problem; simply skim it off, and add more juice. If, however, a lot of fuzzy mold grows, then you should probably throw away your batch and start over.

Other citrus can be fermented, too. Meyer lemons, grapefruit, kumquats, and yuzu are great candidates. Oranges, especially sweet ones, don't work quite as well of their high sugar content. Remember to find pesticide-free citrus, if you can—it is especially important here, because any pesticide on the rind will permeate the preserved fruit.

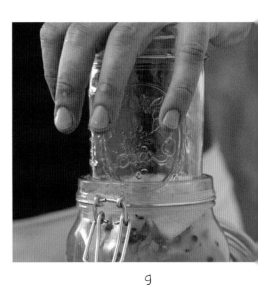

g

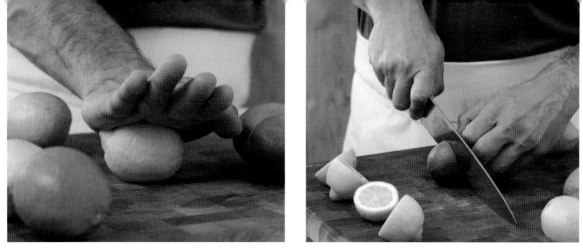

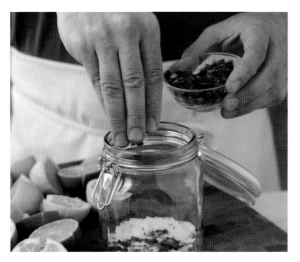

e

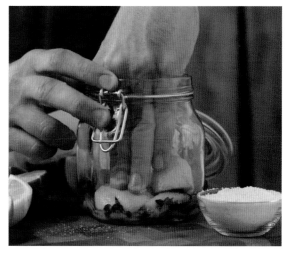

f

## SERVING IDEAS FOR PRESERVED CITRUS

* Mince your preserved lemons and use them in cold salads: cucumber, cucumber-yogurt, tuna, potato. Or chop them fine or purée them and mix them with olive oil for a great salad dressing.

* Slice preserved lemons very thin, and serve them with grilled fish. Or serve them with smoked fish and crème fraîche for a trio of preserved foods!

* Finely mince preserved lemons, combine with freshly ground pepper, and rub under the skin of a whole chicken and inside the body cavity before roasting.

* Use preserved lemon in moderation in a tagine or stew, for a deep citrus flavor.

* In Vietnam, there is a salty drink made with ice, preserved lemon or lime, water or carbonated water, and sugar to taste. The same drink works great with limes, too, or a combination of lemons and limes, or probably with any other citrus. Once you try this, you won't want to go back to regular lemonade.

# PEACH AND PLUM CHUTNEY WITH PRESERVED LIME

Before refrigeration was widespread, and before canning was understood, people used fermentation to preserve all sorts of foods, including chutneys. These foods developed a unique sweet-and-sour flavor.

Today's chutneys are usually preserved with vinegar rather than fermentation. There's nothing really wrong with this, but vinegar-preserved foods don't provide the same health benefits as fermented foods do.

Try this recipe as a side with grilled meats or vegetables: a pork chop, a ham, some swordfish, or a portobello mushroom. You can also mix this chutney into your yogurt for breakfast or a snack, or put it all together in the blender for a great smoothie (add water to thin it out if you like).

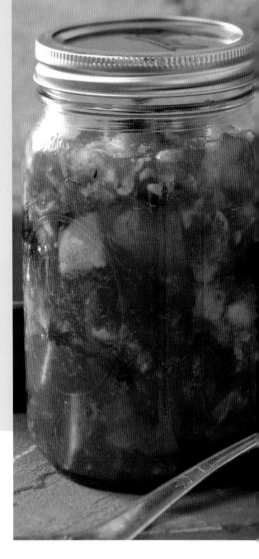

## INGREDIENTS

Several peaches and plums
(approximately 1½ pounds [675 g] total)

A few wedges preserved lime (page 117)

Half a handful chopped walnuts

1 tablespoon (about 6 g) mixed spices,
such as cinnamon, cloves, and peppercorns

2 tablespoons (30 ml) yogurt whey

## EQUIPMENT

Large cutting board (wood is ideal)

Large knife (a chef's knife is ideal)

Large mixing bowl

1-quart (950 ml) mason jar

**Yield: a bit less than
1 quart (950 ml)**

**Prep time: 15 minutes**

**Total time: 4 days**

## PREPARATION

1  Chop the peaches and plums to the desired size, removing the pits (a), (b).

2  Mince the preserved lime (c).

3  Place all the ingredients into the bowl and mix well (d).

4  Transfer the mixture into the jar, and pack down (e). If the juices are insufficient to cover the chutney, add nonchlorinated water until everything is covered, leaving 1 inch (2.5 cm) of headroom.

5  Close the jar lid tightly, and store at room temperature. Open the jar a couple of times a day to relieve pressure.

6  After 2 to 3 days, when the product is slightly fizzy, put it in the refrigerator.

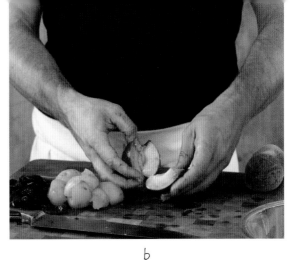

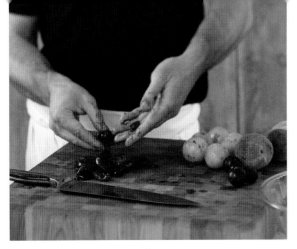

a

b

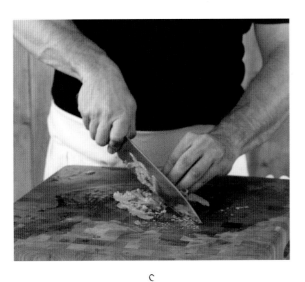

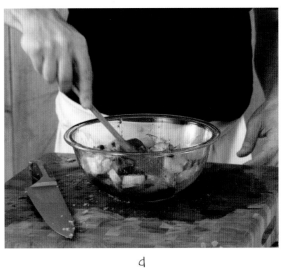

c

d

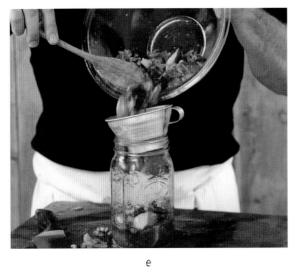

e

## LAB NOTES

* Pressure can build up, so be a little bit careful when opening the jar. You may want to do it over the sink!

* Many variations are possible. One option is to cut apples, pears, or Asian pears into cubes, and use those instead of the softer fruit.

* The chutney will keep in the refrigerator for a month or more.

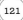

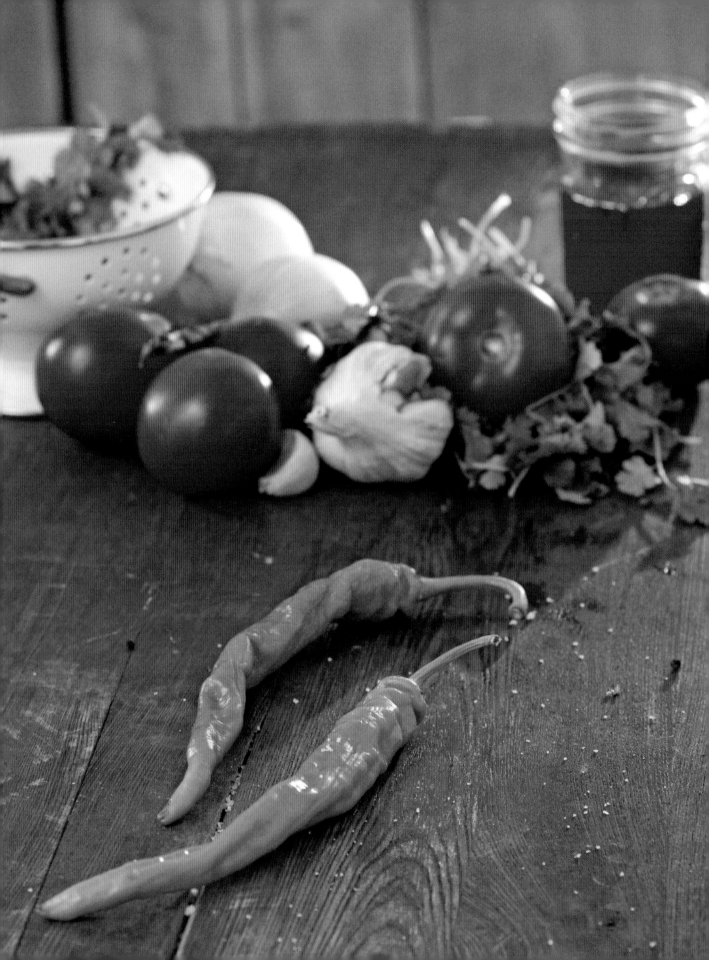

# PICO DE GALLO

*Pico de gallo* literally means "beak of the rooster." It is a condiment made with tomatoes, onions, peppers, herbs, and other flavorings. In North America, it is often referred to as "salsa." I prefer to call it "pico de gallo" because "salsa" is a very general term—it translates as simply "sauce."

This recipe requires sauerkraut juice, ideally from a batch of your own sauerkraut (page 61). If you plan to do a lot of fermenting, it's good to always have some sauerkraut on hand.

Tomato skins and cores can be bitter, so I remove them here. If you prefer to leave them in, that's fine, too.

## INGREDIENTS

6 medium tomatoes

1 large onion

½ bunch cilantro

6 cloves garlic

Hot peppers, to taste

1½ cups (350 ml) sauerkraut juice (page 61), from a batch of sauerkraut you have made (requires prior planning)

Salt and pepper to taste

## EQUIPMENT

Large stockpot

Ice

Mixing bowl

Paring knife

Tongs or a large slotted spoon

Large knife (a chef's knife is ideal)

Large cutting board (wood is ideal)

1-quart (950-ml) mason jar

**Yield: a bit less than 1 quart (950 ml)**

**Prep time: 25 minutes**

**Total time: 3–5 days**

*Recipe continued on page 124*

*Pico de Gallo continued*

## PREPARATION

1 Fill the stockpot with water and bring it to a boil.

2 Prepare an ice bath in the mixing bowl.

3 Cut an "X" on the top of each tomato with the paring knife (a).

4 Using tongs, put the tomatoes in the boiling water for approximately 30 seconds,
all at once or in batches, until the skin starts to peel (b), and then immediately immerse them in the ice bath (c). This will make them easier to peel.

5 Peel the tomatoes (d), remove their cores (e), and use your fingers to remove some or all of the seeds, so that you are left mostly with the flesh.

6 Chop the tomatoes and all of the other solid ingredients, and add them to the mixing bowl (f–n). Add salt and pepper to taste.

7 Pack the mixture into the mason jar (o).

8 Pour the sauerkraut juice over the salsa so that it is covered (p). Use at least 1 cup (235 ml) of the sauerkraut juice, or more as needed to cover up the vegetables. Leave 1 inch (2.5 cm) of headroom.

9 Close the lid and leave the mixture on the counter for 3 to 5 days. Then transfer it to the refrigerator, where it will keep for at least a couple of weeks, and probably much longer.

Pico de gallo is a versatile condiment and flavoring. Have it with an avocado, with sour cream or crème fraîche, or with cheese. Try it on grilled fish, other grilled foods, or with lighter meats. And, of course, you can eat it with tortilla chips!

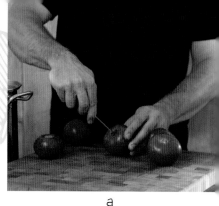

a

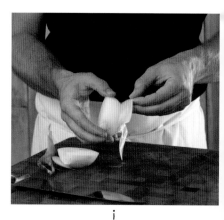

e

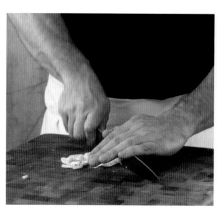

i

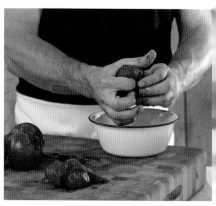

m

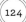

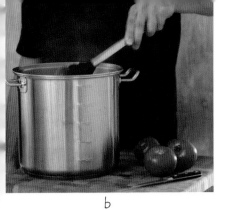

b

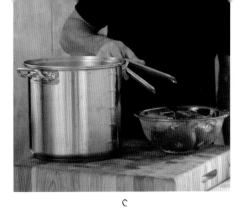

c

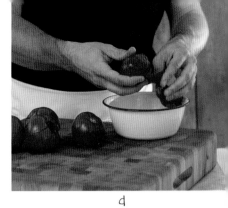

d

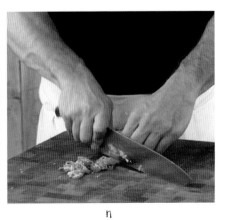

f

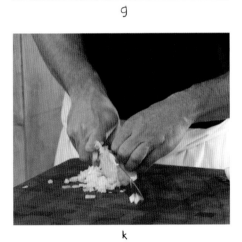

g

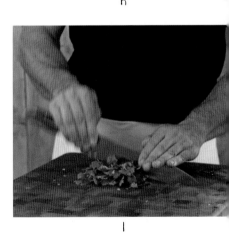

h

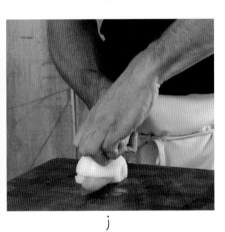

j

k

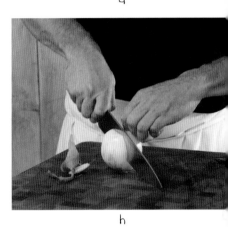

l

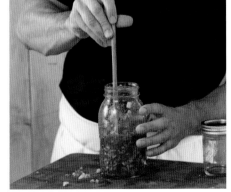

n

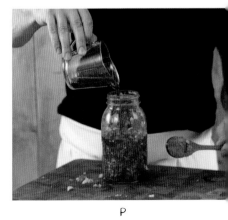

o

p

# CHAPTER 7
# FERMENTED BEVERAGES

THE MOST POPULAR, interesting, and important beverages in the world are fermented.

Before you dismiss this as hyperbole, consider this partial list: coffee, chocolate, and some kinds of tea; every alcoholic beverage, including wine, beer, hard apple cider, mead, sake, and hard liquor; vinegar and kombucha; and dairy beverages based on yogurt and kefir, discussed in chapter 5. All of these are fermented!

COFFEE AND CHOCOLATE ARE BOTH edible in their raw plant state, but their raw states are quite different from their familiar forms, and in order to effect the transformation, they are processed by various methods, including fermentation. Fermentation is used to transform many different foods into beverages, imbuing them with desired qualities such as acidity, alcohol, or additional flavors. In every case, the creation of these drinks relies on the actions of bacteria and/or yeast.

It may not come as a complete surprise that so many important beverages are fermented. Fermentation is one of the oldest and easiest ways in which people can process food, and it remains one of the most intriguing. Evidence of fermented alcoholic beverages stretches back nearly 10,000 years, among diverse peoples.

There is a theory that alcohol and other psychoactive substances were key to the development of human consciousness, to the emergence of our spiritual life, and ultimately to the differentiation of humans from the rest of the animal kingdom. And if we give credence to that theory, then it is worth noting that some species of monkeys have a documented taste for overripe fruit—fruit that has fermented and become alcoholic. We humans need to watch our backs.

Given sufficient time, many beverages will ferment on their own, often with acceptable results. But when we involve ourselves in the process, we can guide it toward a particular goal, further ensuring that the outcome is to our liking.

## HARVEST BUZZ: SOME TRADITIONAL CROPS AND FERMENTED BEVERAGES

| REGION | CROP | BEVERAGE |
| --- | --- | --- |
| Southern Europe | Grapes | Wine |
| Northern Europe | Grain | Beer |
| England and Northeastern U.S. | Apples | Cider |
| Western U.S. | Grapes | Wine |
| Midwestern U.S. | Grain | Beer |
| Latin America | Various | Chicha |
| Southern Africa | Sorghum | Beer |
| East Asia | Rice | Sake and choujiu, soju |

## IS TEA FERMENTED?

Fresh tea leaves go through various transformations to become the tea that we drink; the sequence is different for each type of tea. Black tea and oolong tea undergo a step in the process that is commonly referred to as "fermentation." However, this is not fermentation as we understand the word, because there are no microbes at work. It is more accurately described as oxidation and enzymatic breakdown, or curing, in the absence of microbes. In fact, if microbes do take hold at this stage, the tea can be ruined.

Some green teas are fermented in our sense of the word: they are aged under relatively moist conditions in the open air, and microbes play a role. These are referred to as post-fermented teas. The Chinese tea, *pu-erh*, is one of the best-known post-fermented teas. Teas that have been compressed into blocks for transport and sale are typically post-fermented teas.

And just to make things a little more complicated, it is possible to take brewed, sweetened tea, and ferment *that*, using a specific starter culture; the result is a drink called kombucha, which is discussed later in this chapter (see page 145). Note that in this case the tea is fermented after it has already been brewed into a beverage, unlike chocolate and coffee, which are fermented when they are still in their raw form.

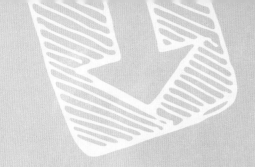

## COFFEE AND CHOCOLATE

Fermentation plays a central role in the processing of coffee and chocolate. In both cases, fermentation helps soften the surrounding pulp so that we can get to the beans. It also plays an important role in developing the flavors of the beans and in helping to preserve them. (There is a stage in the processing of vanilla that is also sometimes referred to as "fermentation," but as with tea, this is enzymatic breakdown and oxidation, and microbes play little or no role.)

Because we rarely take on the fermentation of coffee and chocolate at home, extensive instructions are not provided here.

Alex Whitmore, cofounder of Taza Chocolate in Somerville, Massachusetts, gives us an overview of the role of fermentation in the making of chocolate.

## CACAO FERMENTATION: THE DEVELOPMENT OF FINE CHOCOLATE FLAVORS

**Contributed by Alex Whitmore**, *cofounder of Taza Chocolate*

Most people do not think of chocolate when they are thinking about fermented foods. The fact is, you would have some pretty bad-tasting chocolate if cacao farmers did not take the time to ferment cacao beans before sending them to chocolate makers. All the deep and complex flavors that we enjoy when eating fine chocolate stem from a very unique fermentation process that begins almost the moment the cacao fruit is plucked from the tree.

The source of all chocolate flavors is the fruit of a tree called *Theobroma cacao*. Cacao grows in high-precipitation tropical climates and depends heavily on regular heavy rainfall to produce significant amounts of fruit. The foam-football–shaped fruits contain a slimy, bright white fruit meat that surrounds dark purple seeds (though everyone calls them beans). The beans are extremely bitter and astringent, sort of like eating an apple seed. The fruit, however, is tangy, sweet, and delicious . . . and tastes nothing like chocolate yet.

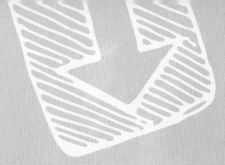

## THE CACAO HARVEST AND NATURAL FERMENTATION

When cacao is harvested, the pods are cracked open, exposing the sweet fruit to the warm tropical air, which is teeming with airborne bacteria and yeasts. The fruit and the beans are scooped out and brought to a centralized fermentation center where they are packed into large wooden boxes. The cacao is left in these boxes for up to a week. During that time the naturally occurring yeasts and bacteria consume the sugars in the fruit, which creates alcohols and other highly acidic compounds that seep into the seeds. These acids break down the bitter compounds and give the resulting cacao beans a deep, nutty, and sometimes fruity or floral flavor.

A very important part of the cacao fermentation process is the generation of heat. The fermentation begins to really heat up after the first day in the boxes, reaching temperatures of up to 112°F (45°C). This heat is critical in breaking down certain bitter compounds in the beans. (The volume of the boxes is very important, too: If the boxes or volume of cacao are too small, the right temperatures cannot be reached, resulting in poor flavor development.)

During an optimum fermentation cycle, the beans are rotated, usually every two days, and oxygen is incorporated into the mass of wet beans. This encourages acetic acid fermentation. Not agitating the beans can result in a lactic fermentation and, as the word implies, a cheesy-tasting chocolate.

Once the beans have been adequately fermented, they are removed from the boxes and spread out to dry in the sun on raised wooden decks. The drying process can take from five to eight days, depending on weather conditions. The beans are then sacked up and shipped to chocolate makers for roasting and grinding.

Amazingly, most cacao farmers never taste the chocolate that their beans end up making; likewise the chocolate maker has little control over this fermen-tation process unless he has a close relation-ship with the cacao producer. For chocolate companies who prize quality and superior flavor, it is imperative that they spend time working with producers to ensure that the fermentation process is right for the chocolate flavor they are looking for.

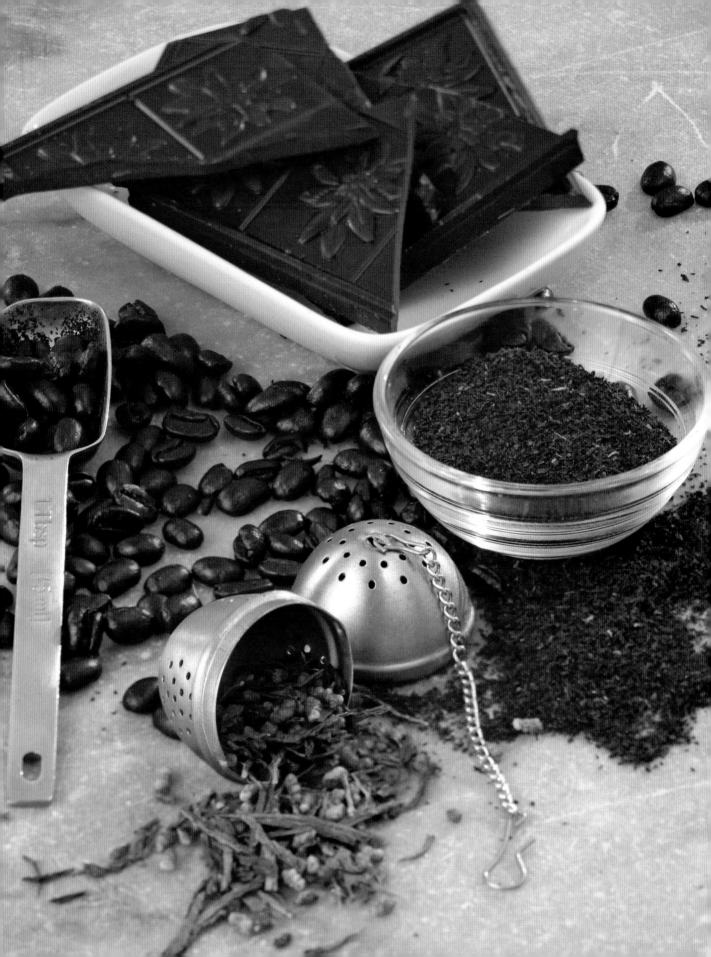

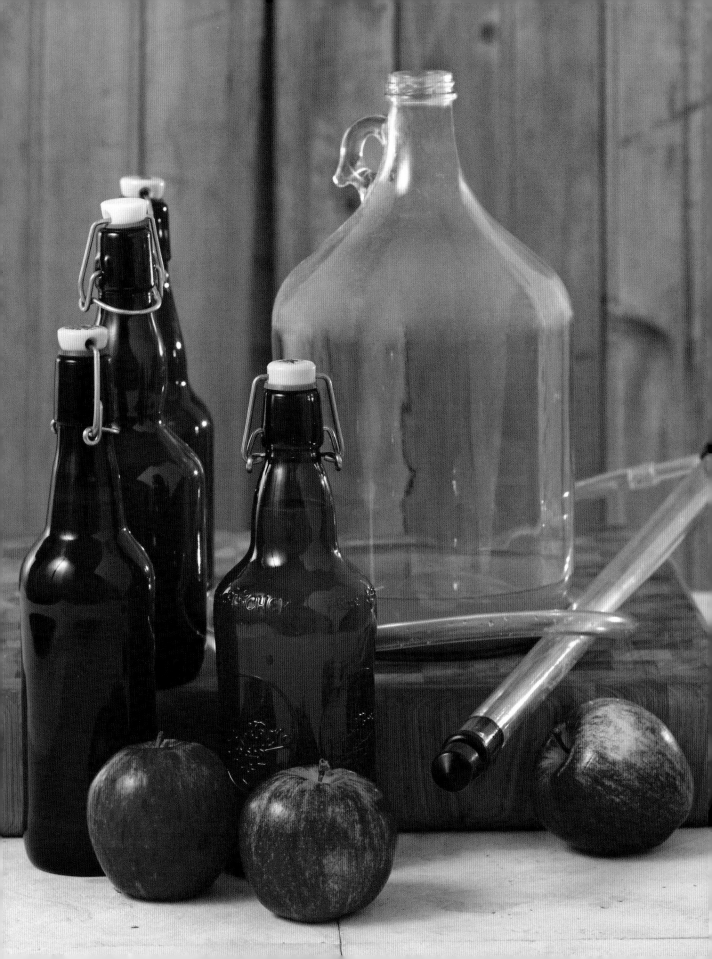

# HARD APPLE CIDER

Hard apple cider is one of the easiest alcoholic beverages to make at home.

If you live in an apple-growing region, you might be able to find fresh, unpasteurized apple cider at a farm or a farm stand. (Organic is best, because nonorganic apples are often heavily treated with pesticides.) If you are fortunate enough to have your own apple trees, even better—use juice from your own apples, especially if they aren't great eating apples which most apples aren't.

If you are able to get unpasteurized apple cider, you may not need this recipe at all. Instead, you can simply let your cider sit, cross your fingers, and within a few weeks, because of natural yeasts, you may have good hard cider, depending on ambient temperatures and other factors.

If you are buying your cider in a store, it has probably been pasteurized. In this case, you will need to use a yeast starter because pasteurization kills the natural yeasts. Using a starter is not a bad thing; it improves the likelihood that your cider will turn out well, and it also gives you a better chance of reproducing your results next time if you come up with a particularly successful cider formula. Even when you start with unpasteurized cider, if you would like to have more control over the process, you can pasteurize your cider yourself, and then ferment it with a starter. In fact, Louis Pasteur's "pasteurization" was originally employed in winemaking.

## YEAST STARTERS

The easiest way to get a yeast cider starter is to buy one. Many kinds are available in home-brewing stores and on the Internet. Some are intended specifically for cider, others for beer, and yet others for wine or champagne or mead.

There are many opinions about which packaged yeast is "best" for making cider. Different yeasts, different ambient temperatures, and different fermentation periods will result in different flavors and different alcohol levels. You can play it safe and buy one that is nominally intended for cider, or you can try another kind. You could even try baking yeast, although the results may not be like the hard cider you're used to.

Another way to get a yeast starter is to capture yeast from your surroundings. You might be able to do this by leaving an open glass of apple cider sitting on the counter, but there's a good chance you won't get what you are looking for—mold might win the day, for instance. A better, although still not surefire, way to get a wild starter is from fruit. If you look closely at some organic fruit—raspberries and grapes, for instance—you will see a white powder on the skin. (You can capture these yeasts as described on page 140.) (It is important that the fruit be organic, because nonorganic fruits are routinely treated with antimicrobial agents. This is done partly to prevent yeast from growing on them!)

*Recipe continued on page 134*

 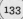

## Hard Apple Cider continued

This recipe is definitely of the "home brew" variety. It is not scientific and will not necessarily make the most sophisticated or refined hard cider, but it is fun and satisfying, provides a good taste of home brewing, and is a good jumping-off point for folks who might go on to do fancier yeast brewing, such as cider-, wine-, mead-, and beermaking, which are quite similar. The door is open to you.

### INGREDIENTS

1 gallon (4 L) fresh, unpasteurized apple cider (or store-bought and home-pasteurized cider)

1 envelope (2 teaspoons, or 8 g) cider yeast, champagne yeast, ale yeast, or wine yeast; or, for a wild starter, 1 cup or so (125 to 150 g) fresh organic raspberries or grapes

### EQUIPMENT

6-quart (6 L) or larger stockpot (optional)

Food thermometer (optional)

1-pint (475-ml) mason jar (optional)

1-gallon (4-L) carboy (if you bought the cider in a 1-gallon [4-L] jug, this will do nicely)

Airlock that fits in the top of the carboy (optional)

Beugel bottles, also known as "Grolsch-type" bottles or swing-top bottles (optional)

Auto-siphon pump and some tubing (optional)

**Yield: 1 gallon (3.8 L)**

**Prep time: 5 minutes or longer**

**Total time: 5–15 days**

## PREPARATION

1 For a wild starter: If you would like to try using a wild starter, put the raspberries or grapes in a pint mason jar, add a cup (250 ml) or so of cider to cover, close the lid, and leave it somewhere warm. Check on it every day. If, after a few days, the contents of the jar have started to get bubbly, then you have successfully captured a yeast starter from your fruit (a)! If a week goes by and nothing has happened, you can try again, or else buy some yeast.

2 Fill the carboy about three-quarters with fresh cider. (If the cider came in the carboy, then pour yourself a glass and drink it to make some space in the bottle!)

3 Add your starter (whether it's a wild starter, as in step 1, or an envelope of yeast) to the carboy of cider (b), cap it, and give the carboy a shake or a swirl (c).

4 Prepare the airlock, if using, and install it into the top of the carboy. If you are using a simple airlock, as pictured, prepare it by removing the cap, half-filling it with water (up to the line) (d), (e), and then replacing the cap (f).

*Recipe continued on page 136*

### APPLE CIDER VERSUS APPLE JUICE

Naming conventions vary from place to place, but in North America, the term "apple cider" is used to denote the unfiltered juice of apples, apple juice refers to the filtered juice of apples, and hard apple cider refers to apple cider that has been fermented with yeast and contains alcohol.

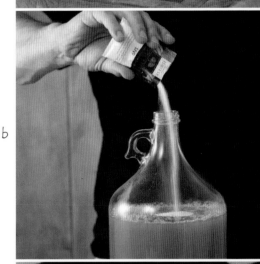

a

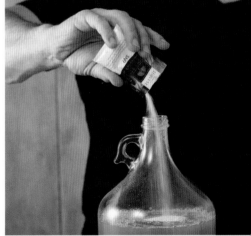

b

c

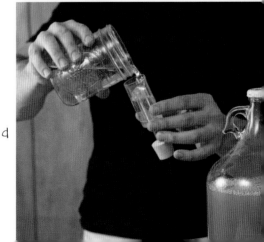

d

## Hard Apple Cider continued

5 Leave the cider somewhere dark and relatively cool for a couple of weeks, or more.

6 Taste your cider periodically. If you'd like to be scientific, you can estimate the alcohol content of the cider by periodically measuring its specific gravity using a hydrometer. Different hydrometers work in different ways; how you take the measurement depends on the particular hydrometer that you buy. In any case, it is not necessary.

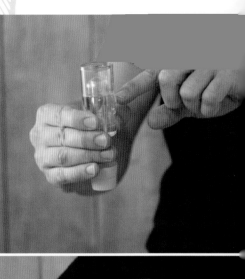

e

7 When you are satisfied with the taste, the level of sweetness, and the alcohol content, you can start to drink the cider, and/or transfer it into swing-top bottles, using an auto-siphon if you have one (g), (h). Sediment will probably have settled out of your cider to the bottom of the carboy; try to avoid disturbing this sediment. (Auto-siphons are designed to avoid disturbing the sediment; they have their inlets some distance above the bottom of the column [i].)

8 If you are moving the cider to bottles, wait until almost all of the sweetness is gone. Too much sweetness means that there is still a substantial amount of sugar left in the cider, which means fermentation will continue in the bottle. If too much fermentation occurs in the sealed bottles, it could result in a buildup of carbon dioxide and, in extreme cases, exploding cider bottles! Swing-top bottles are designed so that the top pops off before the glass breaks, but it is still best to avoid this situation.

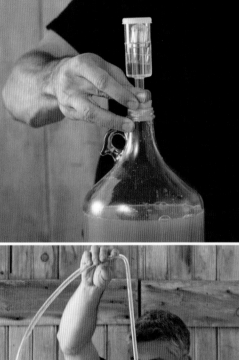

f

Commercial cidermakers and winemakers use chemicals like sodium metabisulfite to kill the yeasts, thus decisively stopping the fermentation. They do this for reasons of economy, process, and consistency, because it would be too costly and unpredictable for them to have bottles exploding here and there. Sodium metabisulfite and similar chemicals can be toxic if not handled properly, so I do not suggest using them at home, although when added to a cider or wine in proper amounts, they may be safe. Part of the beauty of processing your own food is that you can keep an eye on your cider and release some gas from it if necessary, and you don't have to use chemicals to regularize it.

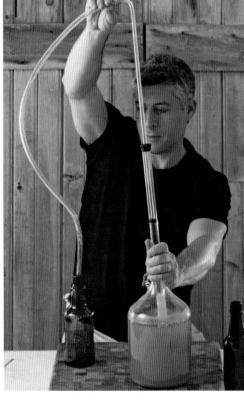

g

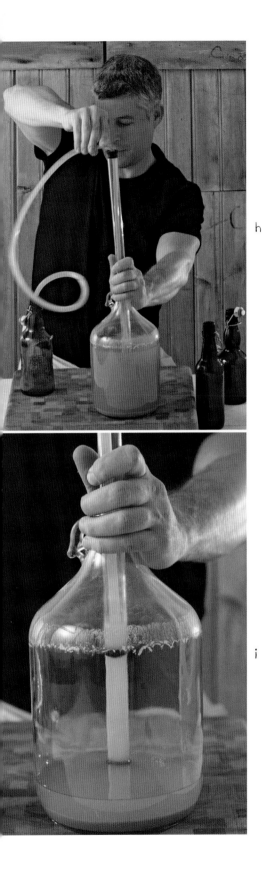

h

i

9   Leaving the cider to age in the sealed bottles will further mellow its flavor; the aging cider may also gain some fizz. Taste your cider every once in a while. If you are getting a lot of carbonation, you might want to relieve some pressure from the bottles (or they might blow their tops!). Putting your cider in the refrigerator will slow the fermentation significantly.

There's no strict rule for how long you can keep cider, just as there's no strict rule for how long you can keep wine. It might be good after a month, or it might be good after years. The only thing I do recommend is that you open a bottle and taste it periodically; when you think it can't get any better, drink the rest! If it starts to taste too sour, you can keep it around for cooking: as a marinade, use it in place of vinegar in recipes, or even open the tops and see if it will turn into a nice vinegar (see 153).

## LAB NOTES

You can use almost any kind of fruit juice (or carrot juice, or any sweet beverage) as a substitute for apple cider in this recipe. This recipe is a basic template for all yeast-fermented beverages, including wine and beer. So please feel free to experiment with other store-bought juices.

Pear juice will result in something not too far off from the apple version; pomegranate juice will give you something quite different. Give it a try with your favorite juice.

Your results will depend on the sugar content and flavor of the original liquid and the type of yeast you use.

And again, if you are going to store it in closed bottles, it is best to wait until most of the sweetness is gone, to avoid excessive buildup of carbon dioxide that might lead to popped tops.

# MEAD

Mead, also known as honey wine, is a fermented beverage made from honey. Pure honey does not invite microbial activity, but when you dilute it with water—two or three parts water to one part honey—the mixture ferments readily into mead.

Mead is one of the most ancient fermented foods. There are some who theorize that it predates grape wine. It has been an important drink in Asia, Europe, and Africa.

As a home brewer, you can prepare mead in much the same way as you prepare cider. Hybrid fermented beverages are also possible: If you ferment a mixture of honey, water, and apple cider, the result is called *cyser* (see Lab Notes, page 139). You can also ferment a mixture of honey, water, and fruit to get a fruit mead.

## INGREDIENTS

2 to 2½ quarts (2 to 2.5 L) nonchlorinated water

1 quart (1.5 kg) honey

1 envelope (2 teaspoons, or 8 g) champagne yeast, ale yeast, or wine yeast; or, for a wild fruit starter, 1 cup or so (125 to 150 g) fresh organic raspberries or grapes

## EQUIPMENT

6-quart (6-L) or larger stockpot

Metal spoon

Food thermometer

1-gallon (4-L) carboy (an empty 1-gallon (3.8-L) apple cider bottle will do nicely)

Airlock that fits into the top of the carboy

Beugel bottles, "Grolsch-type" bottles, or swing-top bottles (optional)

**Yield: 3–3½ quarts (2.8–3.3 L)**

**Prep time: 5 minutes or longer**

**Total time: 5–30 days**

## PREPARATION

1 Put the water into the stockpot and bring it to a boil.

2 Remove from the heat, then add the honey and stir with a metal spoon until well mixed.

3 You have three choices for a starter:

  * Use an envelope of yeast.

  * Make a wild starter with fruit, as in the Hard Apple Cider recipe (step 1 on page 135), but instead of using apple cider use the honey-water mixture.

  * Make a wild starter as in the Hard Apple Cider recipe, but use the honey-water mixture alone, and no fruit.

4 If a significant amount of time has gone by since you combined the water and honey, bring it to a boil again. Regardless, ensure that it is below approximately 100°F (40°C) before proceeding to the next step.

5 Add the starter to the honey-water, stir well, and then pour the mixture into the carboy. Prepare the airlock (as in the Hard Apple Cider recipe, step 4), and insert it into the carboy.

6 Leave the developing mead somewhere dark for a couple weeks. Proceed as for Hard Apple Cider, from step 6.

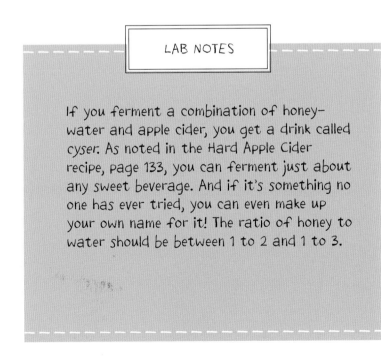

LAB NOTES

If you ferment a combination of honey-water and apple cider, you get a drink called cyser. As noted in the Hard Apple Cider recipe, page 133, you can ferment just about any sweet beverage. And if it's something no one has ever tried, you can even make up your own name for it! The ratio of honey to water should be between 1 to 2 and 1 to 3.

# WINE (IN BRIEF)

Wine is one of the most popular and well-known alcoholic beverages in the world. People have been drinking it for thousands of years. It is the result of yeast fermentation of crushed grapes or grape juice, which converts sugars into alcohol, sometimes followed by controlled bacterial fermentation, which changes the acid profile.

There are a lot of subtleties to making good wine. For instance:

* using particular single varieties of grapes, or a specific blend of different varieties (varietals versus blends);

* separating the skins, meat, and pulp from the juice, or leaving them all together for varying lengths of time (this is part of what accounts for different-colored wines);

* adding particular yeasts (most professionally produced wine is made from very specific yeasts);

* aging wines in barrels made of different materials such as oak, stainless steel, or glass, or in bottles;

* using various additives and filtering agents, to help clarify or preserve the wine;

* blending wines from different batches or years before bottling.

Each of these affects the flavor of the wine, its alcohol level, and how it ages.

When the term *wine* is used on its own, it is understood to mean wine made from grapes. Other fruits and fruit juices can also be used to make fruit wines. "Apple wine" and "hard cider" are more or less synonymous, although one or the other term may be preferred, depending on region.

## WINE AND FERMENTATION

**Corey Beck,** *general manager and director of wine-making at Francis Coppola Winery in Geyserville, California, gives us a short overview of winemaking.*

Put simply, fermentation is the conversion of sugar into alcohol by yeast. Of course, there's much more to the art of making wine than simply adding a bunch of yeast to grape juice. Winemaking starts in the vineyard. Location, weather, soils, rootstock, and clonal selection are all part of winemaking. Once a location is chosen, it takes up to four years before the first grapes will be harvested for wine production. Typically, grapes will be harvested around the 24 to 26 percent sugar range, yielding approximately 14 percent-alcohol wine.

The fermentation process can vary widely depending on the varietal. White grapes are typically loaded directly into a press that squeezes all the juice out of the berries. The juice is then transferred to a stainless steel tank where it will settle for up to 48 hours. The settling process allows for the heavy solids to fall to the bottom of the tank and be removed before fermentation commences. Once the juice has had enough time to settle, the clear juice is racked (transferred) to another tank, and it's there that fermentation begins.

The beauty of fermentation is that there are so many different yeast strains to choose from, each giving the wine unique characteristics. The temperature of the juice when the yeast is added is extremely important. Yeast do not like it when it's too cold; below 50°F (10°C) isn't ideal for them. Most white wines are fermented around 55°F to 60°F (13°C to 16°C); it is at this temperature where most of the wine aromas are being produced from the yeast. Typically, white wine will drop 1 to 2 Brix per day during fermentation, and thus if we start from grape juice with a 24 Brix level, it will take about two weeks for all the sugar to convert into alcohol. (Brix is a measure of the sweetness of a liquid.)

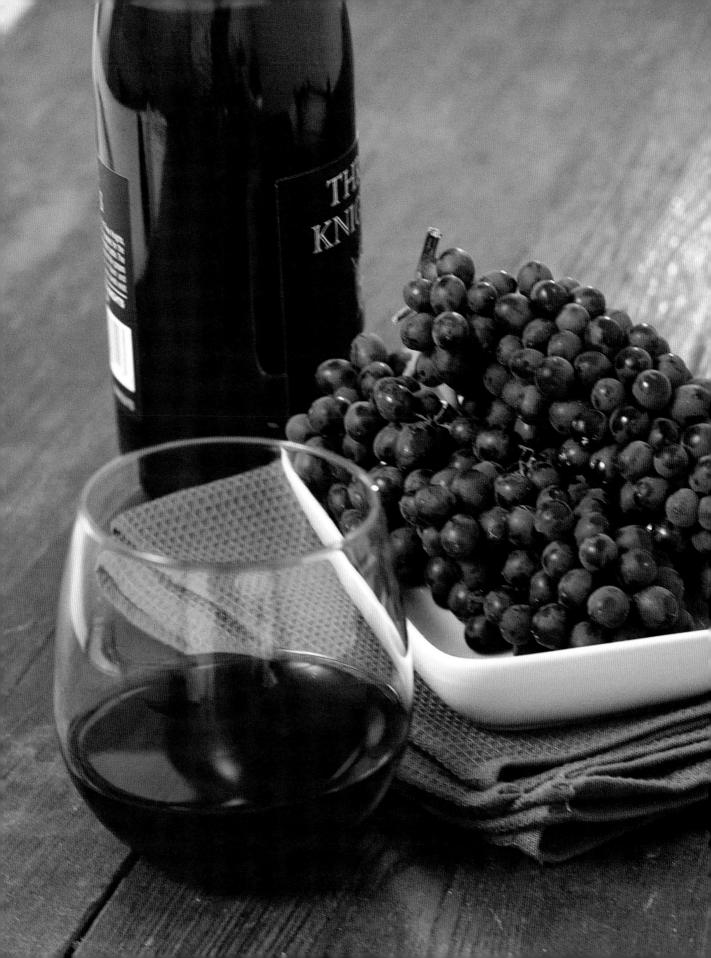

The primary food source in the wine is sugar, and the second is nitrogen, which occurs naturally in grapes. The yeast use these food sources to create three things: heat, carbon dioxide, and alcohol. There are other possible by-products of fermentation; one of them that occurs with Chardonnay grapes is diacetyl, which is the buttery or butterscotch notes in wine. Barrel-fermented wines start off in a tank and then are transferred to barrels to complete the fermentation process. Barrel fermentation gives the wine a richness and vanilla quality that comes from the oak barrels.

Red wine production is somewhat different because the fermentation takes place on the skins of the grapes. Red grapes have clear juice, and the color comes from the pigment in the skins. The grapes are crushed, and the juice and skins are combined in a tank together. Once everything is safely in the tank, yeast are added and fermentation begins. Unlike white wine fermentation, red wine production does best at warmer temperatures, closer to 80°F (30°C). The higher temperatures help extract the color from the red grape skins. Because the temperatures are higher, the yeast are more active and the Brix drop is 4 to 5 per day, so fermentation can be complete in seven days or so. Another compound being extracted from the skins during the fermentation is tannin, which is the flavor building block for red wines. Tannin is what you feel in the sides of your mouth after you drink a Cabernet Sauvignon. Varietals such as Pinot Noir have less tannin, and thus are softer and more approachable at an earlier age. Cabernet Sauvignon has some of the most tannin out of all varietals, and thus takes longer to open up, but will age for years.

Once the fermentation is complete, the pomace is transferred to a press where the remaining juice is squeezed out of the skins. Once the skins have been squeezed they are disposed of and used for compost or fertilizer that goes back to the vineyard. The wine pressed from the red skins will then be transferred to barrels for aging.

# BEER AND KVASS (IN BRIEF)

Beer is another ancient fermented alcoholic beverage and is the most popular alcoholic beverage in the world. Instead of starting from fruit juice or honey, beer starts from grain of some sort, generally barley but sometimes corn, rice, sorghum, millet, or cassava.

The grain undergoes a process known as malting, during which it is soaked until it begins to sprout and is then dried. Malting creates enzymes that start to convert the starches in the grain into sugars. The malted grains are then milled, flavored, and mixed with hot water. Various substances, principally and very commonly hops, may be added along the way for flavor. The result is a sweet liquid called wort, which is then fermented in roughly the same manner as apple juice or grape juice.

Here are some beer variations from around the world:

In South America, *cauim* and related beverages are made from manioc (cassava). In place of the malting process, these cassava-based beers start by having people chew and spit out the manioc; enzymes in their saliva convert the starches into sugar.

Russian *kvass* (or bread kvass) is a traditional, low-alcohol, beer-like drink that is made by soaking stale rye bread and fermenting it with yeast.

Ethiopian *tella* is made in much the same way as traditional European beers.

There are copious beermaking resources on the Internet, as well as many beer brewers who love to share their interest. In particular, if you would like to try your hand at brewing beer, find a store specializing in home brewing, either in your neighborhood or on the web. In such a store, you will find all of the equipment and ingredients you need, and more than likely a few people who are extremely enthusiastic about brewing beer and eager to share their knowledge and experience with you. There are also numerous books and magazines on the subject.

## SAKE

Sake is a rice-based Japanese fermented beverage. It is unusual among popular fermented beverages in that it requires the use of a fungus (most fermented beverages rely only on yeasts and/or bacteria). Sake is made by polishing rice, cooking it, and inoculating it with a specific mold known as *kōji*, which helps convert the rice starch into sugar. While this conversion is happening, yeast is added as well, so that the sugars are converted into alcohol simultaneously. As fermentation progresses, water, rice, and *kōji* are added. Finally, the solids are pressed and the liquid is racked (poured off into a new container); it may be filtered; and finally it is bottled.

Sake makers, like producers of wine and beer, have come up with numerous refinements that lead to better results. There are also many variations on the basic sake template, resulting in a huge variety of possible flavors and qualities.

Traditional sake making involves many steps and is trickier than making some other fermented beverages. So while it's important to know where sake fits into the fermented foods firmament, it is not necessarily the best fermentation project for the novice to attempt at home, and I do not offer instructions for it in this book.

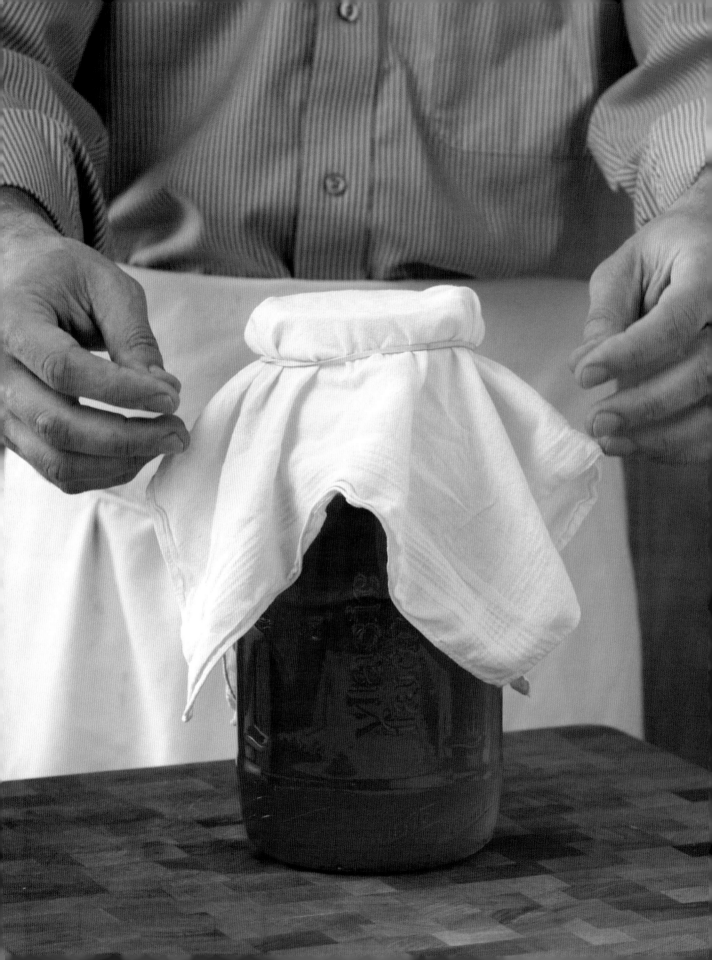

# KOMBUCHA

Kombucha, also known as "tea kvass," is a fermented beverage that typically contains very little alcohol, so it is generally considered nonalcoholic. Kombucha is not nearly as universal as wine and beer, and its history is not as well understood. Despite this, or perhaps because of it, kombucha has developed pockets of dedicated followers.

Current and former kombucha fans include characters as diverse as Aleksandr Solzhenitsyn, Ronald Reagan, and Madonna. Kombucha's healing properties have been widely discussed and pondered. Partly because there is not a large global market for kombucha and not as much formal research has been done into its biochemistry. But it contains a variety of bacteria, healthy yeasts, and enzymes, like many other fermented foods, so it has similar benefits. Recent research does suggest that kombucha's glucaric acid may be an effective liver tonic, helping the liver eliminate waste (including waste from chemotherapy), and that kombucha microbes may help the gut maintain a good balance of bacteria.

## THE KOMBUCHA MOTHER: SCOBY

The cellulosic mat known as the "mother," "SCOBY," or "tea mushroom" is kombucha's signature trait. In appearance and texture it resembles a flat piece of abalone or squid. SCOBY is an acronym for "Symbiotic Colony of Bacteria and Yeast." This mat is both the by-product of kombucha fermentation and the medium on which the bacteria and yeast live. Sometimes the SCOBY is called a "mushroom"; this is inaccurate. To get started making kombucha, you will want to find a SCOBY and some kombucha liquid. These can be bought over the Internet, but depending on where you live, you may be able to find someone giving them away near you, because every time you make a batch of kombucha, a new SCOBY forms.

### SCOBY FROM SCRATCH

If you can't find a kombucha SCOBY, but you have access to kombucha in your supermarket, you can try creating a SCOBY by starting from a bottle. Follow the recipe here, use your bottle of kombucha as the starter, and skip the part about the SCOBY. It may take substantially longer than 5 to 15 days, and it might simply not work. It might work, however, and if you find yourself with a SCOBY, you can make more (and more) kombucha for yourself from that one purchase.

*Recipe continued on page 146*

## Kombucha continued

Besides the SCOBY, kombucha's ingredients are very simple: water, tea, and sugar. As always, use chlorine-free water. If you boil tap water for 10 or 15 minutes, most of the chlorine will evaporate. For more information about water, see page 47.

Plain, organic black, oolong, or green tea is the best choice. The spices used in flavored teas can sometimes interfere with the bacteria and yeast; for instance, bergamot, used in Earl Grey tea, has antimicrobial properties. Not surprisingly, the preservatives and chemicals used on nonorganic tea can also have antimicrobial properties.

Finally, any kind of sugar is fine to use, although if you are seeking to avoid GMOs (see page 46), you may want to skip beet sugar, which is often GM, and get cane sugar, which is not. And if you would like to get some extra trace minerals, turbinado sugar is excellent as is honey. Don't worry about the large amounts of sugar involved in the making of kombucha; most or almost all of the sugar gets metabolized by the SCOBY and converted into acids. For exactly this reason, artificial and/or noncaloric sweeteners will not work; the SCOBY will only eat actual sugar.

The more sour the kombucha, the more sugar that has been converted.

INGREDIENTS

Approximately 2 quarts (2 L) noncholorinated water

2 teaspoons (10 g) *plain* black, oolong, or green tea (or a combination), loose or in bags (tea bags are typically 2 to 4 g each)

¾ cup (150 g) sugar

¾ cup (175 ml) kombucha starter, from a previous, recent batch

1 piece kombucha "mother" (at least several square inches [2.5 cm] in area), also known as SCOBY

**Yield: 2 quarts (2 L)**

**Prep time: 20 minutes**

**Total time: 5–15 days**

## EQUIPMENT

4-quart (4-L) saucepan with lid

Clean 3-quart (3-L) or larger glass jar or jug (clean it with boiling water)

Clean metal spoon (clean it with boiling water)

Clean white handkerchief or towel and a rubber band that can cover the top of the jug or jar

Large ladle

4 or 5 mason jars (1 pint, or 475 ml each) for storing the finished kombucha

*Recipe continued on page 148*

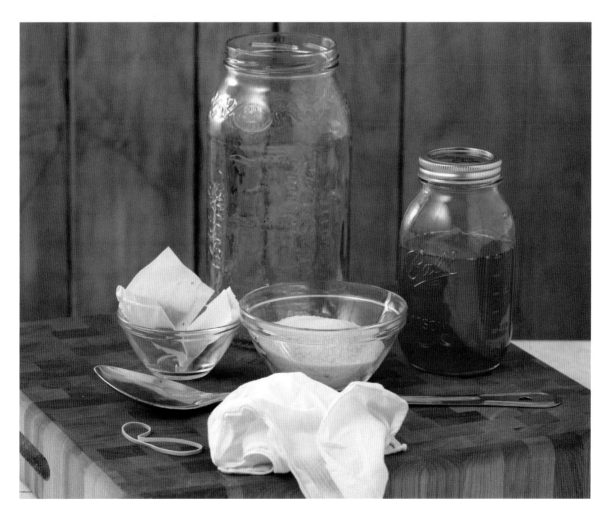

EQUIPMENT AND INGREDIENTS FOR MAKING KOMBUCHA

## PREPARATION

1 Put the water in the saucepan and bring it to a boil. Turn off the heat.

2 Place the tea in a large jar, pour the boiling water over it (a), put the lid on, let the mixture steep for 10 to 15 minutes, and remove the tea (by removing the bags, or by straining if the tea is loose).

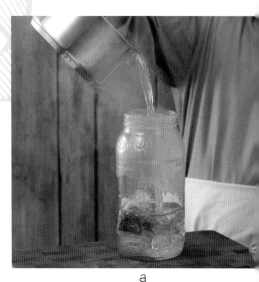

a

3 Add the sugar to the brewed tea (b), and stir with a metal spoon until it is dissolved. Put the lid back on, and let the mixture cool to approximately room temperature.

4 Add half the kombucha starter to the glass jug, and then add the "mother" (c ) and the remainder of the starter (d). (The "mother" may float or sink; it's okay either way.)

5 Cover the top of the jug with the handkerchief and rubber band to keep flies and other foreign objects out (e). Carefully move it somewhere that will maintain warm room temperature, away from direct light.

6 After 5 days, start tasting your kombucha with a very clean spoon (you can rinse the spoon in boiling water before using it). The brew should be tart but not unpleasantly sour. If it is still sweet, let it brew for another day or two, then taste it again.

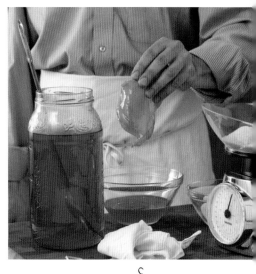

c

7 When you are happy with your kombucha, pour or ladle most of it into mason jars, leaving a bit of room at the top of each. Store them at a cool room temperature or in the refrigerator. Reserve some of the kombucha plus the "mother," and use these to start your next batch.

8 If you like, you can give some of your extra "mother" and some starter to a friend. Wash your hands carefully, pick up the "mother," cut it with a clean knife if necessary, and put it in a jar with some liquid. Keep for yourself at least as much "mother" as you used in your previous batch. If your next batch will be larger, then keep more.

To brew a batch that's bigger than 2 quarts (2 L), scale the recipe accordingly. So for each quart (950 ml) of water, you will use 6 tablespoons (80 g) sugar, 1 teaspoon (5 g) loose tea (or two teabags), and 6 tablespoons (90 ml) starter liquid, plus, of course, your SCOBY.

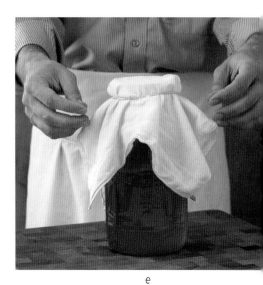

e

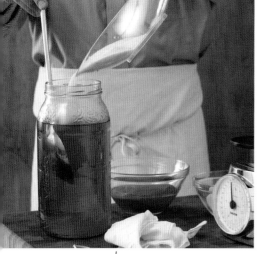

b

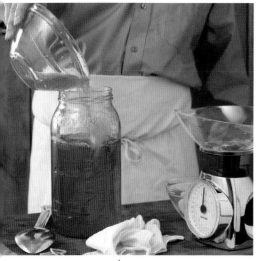

d

If you buy kombucha from the store, you can save the bottles and use them for storing your own homemade kombucha. The jars tend to be 12 to 16 ounces (355 to 475 ml) and made of thick glass, so they're suitable for this application.

If you don't want to start your next batch immediately, you can store your kombucha starter and "mother" in a jar in the refrigerator for a couple of months.

The longer you store your finished, bottled kombucha at room temperature, the more carbonation you may get.

If you use plain black, oolong, or green tea (or a combination), it is possible to maintain a kombucha SCOBY lineage indefinitely. But if you would like to experiment with using a kombucha starter to ferment herbal teas, flavored teas, barley tea, fruit juice, and so on, feel free. In this case, it is always wise to keep some extra tea-only starter and "mother" on hand and to continue brewing them using plain tea, so that there is a fallback if your experimental strain eventually fails.

Exotically flavored kombuchas are popular and are available in many stores. Strawberry, mango, ginger, blueberry, and spirulina all find their way into kombucha. If you want to make flavored kombucha at home, purée your flavorings and add them to jars of finished kombucha. Store these flavored kombuchas on a shelf for a while before refrigerating, to get carbonation and a more thorough blending of flavors. Adding the flavorings at the end is better than adding them during brewing. Some flavorings attract the wrong sorts of microbes if added too soon; others, like ginger, have antimicrobial properties that could potentially affect fermentation.

# KOMBUCHA MOTHER: AN OWNER'S MANUAL

--------------------------------

**by Annabelle Ho,** *author of the blog Kombucha Fuel,*
*www.kombuchafuel.com*

Every time you brew a batch of kombucha, a new kombucha mother—the SCOBY— typically forms on the surface. Ideally, a healthy kombucha mushroom is a cream-colored, ⅛" – ¼" -thick pancake. If your kombucha culture does not fit this description, do not worry! Many factors, such as low and inconsistent brewing temperatures, different brewing environments, brewing duration, and more, can affect the kombucha mushroom.

Younger mushrooms tend to have a light, creamy color, which develops into a darker brown color as the cultures age. An incompletely formed mushroom or a SCOBY with varied thicknesses is perfectly fine to use for most individuals' home-brewing purposes. In addition, because the kombucha mushroom grows on the surface of the container that it ferments in, SCOBYs will always take on the shape of the container.

Younger mushrooms tend to perform (or ferment) better than older ones do. Once you've grown a good, young mushroom, you can store the older one in the refrigerator as a backup or give it to friends.

If you don't see a new mother forming on the surface of your kombucha, here are some tips:

* **Sleeping SCOBY:** Was your SCOBY stored in the fridge? Kombucha mushrooms go "dormant" in the fridge and may need a few cycles to get fully back into gear. Wait a few cycles to see whether new SCOBYs begin forming.

* **Conjoined SCOBY:** Is your kombucha mother sitting on the surface of the kombucha as it brews, and is it getting thicker? If it is, then there's a good chance that the new mushroom is forming right on top of the old one, and the two mushrooms are indistinguishable from each other.

* **Room to breathe:** Be sure to leave a few inches (cm) of air space at the surface of the fermentation vessel to allow room for the baby SCOBY to grow.

* **Shelve the soap:** Avoid cleaning your brewing vessel and equipment with antibacterial soap because SCOBYs contain bacteria. Distilled white vinegar can be used to clean your kombucha equipment and brewing vessel prior to use instead.

* **Caution: hot.** Don't add SCOBYs to hot or warm tea because hot temperatures can kill the culture. Add SCOBYs to sweetened tea that is at room temperature.

* **No smoking!** Avoid brewing in environments where there is smoke (including smoke from cooking), pollen, or toxic fumes such as from paints or solvents.

* **Stay out of the sun:** Do not brew on a windowsill where there is direct sunlight.

* **Stay still:** Keep your fermentation vessel in an undisturbed spot. Every time you move the fermentation vessel while it is brewing, the new baby mushroom begins forming all over again.

* **Keep it simple:** Use only plain, unflavored, and raw kombucha as starter (from the previous batch or purchased from a store). Remember to avoid any foreign additions and flavors when brewing kombucha (such as herbs, spices, certain types of tea, etc.) and to only add these to finished kombucha.

* **Stay sweet:** Ensure that your sweetener contains some form of sugar in either a dry or a crystalline form, such as evaporated cane juice or Sucanat, or in a liquid form, such as honey. Stevia and artificial sweeteners do not provide the necessary food for the yeasts.

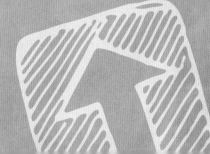

* **Age matters:** The ability for SCOBYs to ferment the tea and to produce new babies tends to decrease as they age. Older SCOBYs are darker brown in color while younger SCOBYs typically have a creamy, white color.

## Growing a Thick Kombucha Mushroom

Because the kombucha may be ready to drink before a well-formed kombucha mushroom fully develops, growing a nice, thick kombucha mushroom is not always synonymous with brewing delicious kombucha. However, having a thick SCOBY can be advantageous as thicker mushrooms tend to ferment the tea more effectively, to a certain extent. A ⅛" – ¼" -thick mushroom is healthy.

To grow a thick kombucha mother, you can put some unflavored and raw kombucha in a clean glass jar, cover it with a breathable cloth, and secure the cloth with a rubber band. Let it sit for a few weeks in a warm, undisturbed spot until a thick mother grows and develops. Alternatively, allow one of your kombucha brews to ferment for a prolonged period of time until a thick SCOBY forms. The process may take several weeks.

The kombucha will become strong, sour, and acidic if it has been fermenting for a long time, which you may not want to drink. This tea can be used as starter tea, however.

## Brewing Rate

There are two significant factors that can affect the rate of the brewing process:

* **Temperature:** Kombucha brews ideally at around 75°F–85°F (25°C–30°C). Kombucha can brew at temperatures slightly above and below that range. However, if the temperature is lower than mid 60°F (around 18°C), use something to increase the temperature of your brew, such as a seedling mat.

* **The amount of starter tea used:** Typically it is recommended to use around 10 to 20 percent starter tea in the overall brew. During the warmer months, you can use closer to 10 percent of starter tea, because fermentation will be faster. In the colder months, use closer to 20 percent starter tea to help get the fermentation process going.

## SCOBY Storage: Refrigerating the Kombucha Mushroom

Refrigerating the kombucha mushroom is usually the easiest method for SCOBY storage between batches. Store the kombucha mushroom in a glass jar with some unflavored kombucha tea. Or, kick-start the brewing process for several days to get the pH level down, and refrigerate the mushroom in its brewing container. This will make the kombucha culture "dormant." It won't be completely inactive, but the SCOBY will be active at a very slow rate, and it can keep this way for months. Keep the lid closed only loosely, so that carbon dioxide doesn't build up and pop the top off.

Consider giving the SCOBY some fresh air and oxygen by opening the lid every now and then. If the kombucha mushroom is in the refrigerator for several weeks or more, it is recommended to add some sweet tea to it every now and then, to give the yeasts additional sugars to feed on. If you would like to resume brewing with a mushroom that has been stored in the refrigerator, allow the SCOBY stored in kombucha to warm up to room temperature overnight before use. When you begin brewing again, it may also take a few cycles for the SCOBY to kick back into full gear.

## Mold

When kombucha is brewed properly and with good kitchen sanitation, the chance of mold contamination is low, because kombucha's anti-microbial properties and acidic pH protect it. If mold does appear, it will be on the top of the SCOBY, and will look fuzzy, like the mold on food and bread. When this happens, the SCOBY and the batch of kombucha should be thrown out, to be safe.

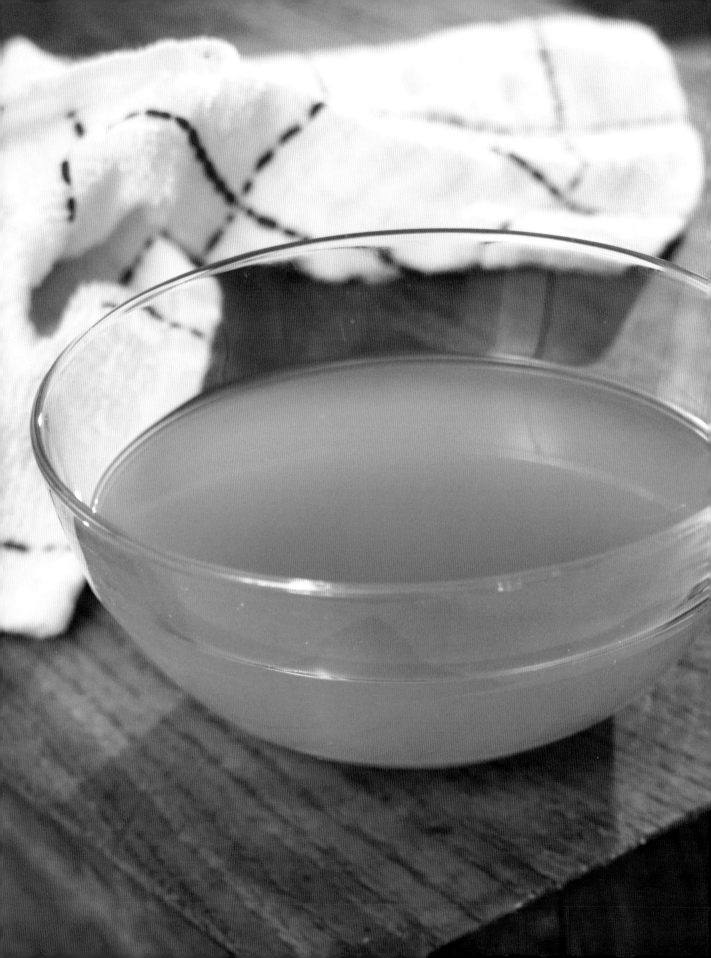

# VINEGAR

Vinegar is traditionally made by the further fermentation of an alcoholic liquid: bacteria convert the alcohol into acetic acid. These bacteria can either be wild, finding the liquid on their own, or they can be added by us. As vinegar ferments, a sort of slime can form. This slime is analogous to the mat that forms during the brewing of kombucha (see page 145), and is similarly called the "mother" or "mother of vinegar." Sometimes this is filtered out of the vinegar before use, and sometimes vinegar is pasteurized prior to sale or distribution to prevent the formation of more mother.

Vinegar is typically not drunk straight. It is sometimes mixed with water and perhaps a sweetener or some herbs—sometimes as a digestive or liver tonic, or for medicinal purposes. Raw vinegars have more tonic properties than pasteurized ones because of the live bacteria, and in fact, an ounce (30 ml) or so of raw apple cider vinegar, diluted with water, is recommended by some as an excellent drink to have first thing in the morning.

Vinegar's widest application these days is as a recipe ingredient. Vinegar has many culinary uses. Because of its high acidity, it is useful and effective for preserving food. It also provides a sharp or sour flavor for dishes that would otherwise lack bite. It is popular with leafy vegetables to offset their sometimes bitter flavor; with meats it was used along with spices before refrigeration to mask rancidity, and where it can also help prevent the palate from being overwhelmed by fat; and with sweet foods.

If you would like to make vinegar at home, wine and hard cider are good starting points. Vinegar, like kombucha, needs some air to ferment; try using an open crock with a cloth over it, stored in a dark place. If you simply add wine or hard cider to a crock and let it stand, you may get good vinegar, but keep in mind that commercially sold wine and cider may contain preservatives, and they may not turn into very good vinegar on their own. Even if it turns into good vinegar, it may take a long time. To help things along, use a starter. You may be able to get a vinegar starter from a friend; otherwise, you can try using some raw apple cider vinegar, which is available in many supermarkets. One part starter in ten or one in twenty should be enough to get things going.

*Recipe continued on page 154*

APPLE CIDER VINEGAR

Vinegar continued

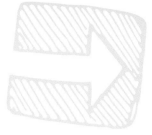

## INGREDIENTS

1 quart (950 ml) wine, apple cider, or other fermented beverage

¼ cup (60 ml) vinegar from a previous batch, or some store-bought raw apple cider vinegar, to use as starter (optional)

## EQUIPMENT

Carboy, bottle, crock, or jar, ideally dark-colored glass and definitely lead-free

Handkerchief or towel with which to cover the container; you want to keep foreign matter out but allow the vinegar to breathe

Rubber band or piece of string

Yield: 1 quart (946 ml), to start

Prep time: Minimal

Total time: Months; varies

## PREPARATION

1 Pour your wine or cider into the vessel.

2 Add the starter, if using—roughly 1 tablespoon (15 ml) for every cup (250 ml) of liquid, or ¼ cup (60 ml) starter per quart (950 ml) of liquid.

3 Cover with the cloth, fasten with the rubber band or string, leave in a dark place, and wait. Be patient. Taste the vinegar occasionally to monitor fermentation, but it will likely take one or two months to become fully sour.

Unfinished bottles of wine are great for this recipe. Once you have some vinegar in progress, you can add to it wine from any unfinished bottles that linger in your kitchen.

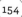

It is important to use a nonreactive vessel for making vinegar. Dark glass is a safe choice. A dark "jug wine" bottle is ideal. If you are using a crock, be very sure that its glazing is stable and contains no lead.

In most recipes calling for vinegar, you can use incompletely fermented vinegar, somewhere between wine (or cider) and vinegar. A little alcohol in your salad dressing shouldn't be a problem—and if you are going to be cooking your vinegar anyway, whatever residual alcohol there is will likely boil off. But, if you or any of your guests are sensitive to alcohol, you may want to stick to commercially produced vinegar, especially if you will be consuming it raw, such as in a salad dressing.

Also, if you are canning, you are better off using commercially produced vinegar. Canning recipes depend on specific levels of acidity in order to be safe. The acidity of commercial vinegar is measured, regulated, and standardized; when you see a bottle of vinegar that is labeled as 5 percent, for instance, this corresponds to a pH level of slightly below 3. When you make vinegar at home, you don't always know how acidic it is. You can buy a kit to measure the acidity of your home-brewed vinegar, but, when in doubt, use standardized vinegar.

# OTHER CULTURED BEVERAGES

The ancestors of modern sodas were naturally fermented drinks. These traditional beverages typically used decoctions or infusions of medicinal roots, leaves, nuts, or barks as their base, possibly with the addition of some fruit and perhaps a stimulant. Their origins are evident if you look closely at the names of the drinks: "root beer," "ginger ale," "coca," and "cola." They would have been fermented through the addition of sugar and bacterial starter culture, resulting in a slightly sweet, slightly sour, low- or no-alcohol drink containing trace minerals and beneficial bacteria.

The carbon dioxide and phosphoric acid added to today's sodas are meant to evoke the carbonation and acidity that are the natural by-products of fermentation in traditional fermented drinks. Unfortunately, modern sodas have none of the health benefits of traditional fermented drinks, contain far more sugar, and also contain colorings and additives that can be toxic. Consumption of phosphoric acid, for instance, has been shown to lower bone density and cause kidney problems.

# GINGER ALE

It is easy to make fermented versions of drinks like root beer and ginger ale, or to invent your own fermented soft drinks, at home. The ingredients are simple: water, extracts, and flavorings of your choice, sugar, and a starter. Generally, you can make a fermented soda using any kind of herbal extract or tea as a base. Ginger ale is a good place to start. (For root beer, see "Root Variations," page 159.)

## INGREDIENTS

3 to 4 inches (7.5 to 10 cm) ginger root

1 gallon (4 L)  nonchlorinated water

1½ cups (300 g) sugar

½ to 1 cup (125 to 250 ml) yogurt whey (see 102), as starter

## EQUIPMENT

Box grater or rasp

Stockpot

Large spoon

Carboy with either a tight-fitting cap or an airlock

Several smaller bottles or jars: swing-top bottles, old kombucha bottles, old glass soda bottles, or 1-pint (475-ml) mason jars

**Yield: 1 gallon (3.8 L)**

**Prep time: 30 minutes**

**Total time: 3–7 days**

## PREPARATION

1 Peel and grate the ginger. The edge of a spoon is an excellent instrument for peeling ginger.

2 Add the ginger and the water to the stockpot and bring to a boil. Continue to boil for a couple of minutes. You now have ginger "tea." (It is not tea in the technical sense, because it is not made from the tea plant *Camellia sinensis*.)

3 Remove from the heat, add the sugar, and stir until dissolved.

4   Allow to cool to warm room temperature.

5   Add the whey starter to the sweetened tea.

6   Pour the mixture into the carboy.

7   Prepare the airlock, and install it in the carboy. (If you are not using an airlock, put the cap on, and then open it to "burp" the carboy at least a couple of times a day for the first few days.)

8   Keep the carboy somewhere at room temperature, or a little cooler, for a few days.

9   Your ginger ale should get fizzy in a few days. After a few more days, when the fizz is subsiding, it may be time to bottle it. Pour it into your smaller bottles or jars, and fill them almost to the top, leaving only a little room. Leave these bottles out at room temperature for a few more days, then put them somewhere cool or in the refrigerator.

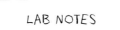

## LAB NOTES

The trick is to bottle your ginger ale while it is still actively fermenting, so that you will trap some carbonation in your bottles—but not so soon that you get too much carbonation for your bottles to contain!

Timing varies greatly, depending on the ambient temperature, but also depending on the activity level of your whey, which is hard to predict. Be prepared for your ginger ale to behave differently every time.

Whey is the easiest starter to use. Anything else that would work for making lacto-fermented sauerkraut (Basic Sauerkraut, page 61) would also work here, although depending on what kind of soft drink you are making, sauerkraut juice may not be the tastiest choice of starter. If you do use sauerkraut juice, be aware that it is not as powerful a starter as whey, so you will need to use more—closer to 1 cup (250 ml) of juice per gallon (4 L) of water.

You can add other seasonings to your ginger ale, including salt, lemon juice, or even fruit juice. Play around with the proportions to suit your taste. You can cut open a vanilla pod, add it to the water, and boil it with the ginger. Most other seasonings and flavorings should be added at the beginning. If you are adding vanilla extract, however, add it at the end.

## FERMENTED VEGETABLE JUICE ("KVASS")

You can easily make a cultured beverage out of beet juice, carrot juice, or any other sort of vegetable juice, following the same general format as with the other beverages in this chapter. If you are using juices with relatively high sugar content, like beet or carrot, you may not need to add any sugar; other juices may fare better if you add some sugar or fruit.

Liquid from sauerkraut, or from other fermented vegetables, is a good choice when making fermented vegetable juice because the flavors are likely to work well together.

Fresh juice, extracted using a juicer, will probably yield a tastier, healthier drink than pasteurized, bottled juice from the store—but don't let that stop you from experimenting with what is available to you.

The general model is the same as in the Ginger Ale recipe on page 156.

## WATER KEFIR

You can buy something called a "water kefir," or *tibicos*, culture. It is similar to dairy kefir (and to kombucha) in that it is a colony of yeast and bacteria that can be used to ferment beverages. It is different from a dairy kefir in that it can ferment a wider variety of beverages and is intended primarily for making fermented *nondairy* beverages. A water kefir starter will give you a different set of microbes from what you'd get with a lacto-fermentation starter like whey or sauerkraut juice because the water kefir starter contains yeast as well as bacteria.

Making a fermented beverage using the water kefir starter is similar to making a beverage using the Ginger Ale recipe, page 156. If you are aiming to get a fizzy end product, the choice of when to bottle it is important. Also be aware that you will want to strain your beverage as you are bottling it because you will want to recover the water kefir starter to use it again! Water kefir starters can be bought online.

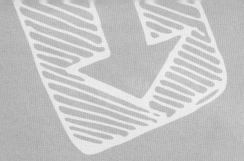

# TIME TO EXPERIMENT

You are now equipped to perform several different kinds of fermentation on whatever (sweet) liquid you choose, using a variety of starters:

* yeast

* whey

* juice from fermented vegetables

* kombucha starter

* water kefir starter

As an experiment, why not gather a bunch of mason jars, choose a handful of juices or sweet liquids, and try each of a few different starters in each of the different liquids, to see how they all come out? Some will be better than others, and some might not be very good; some will take longer than others, and some might not really work at all. But there is no need to worry about "failure," because this is an experiment. Who knows—maybe you will discover your new favorite drink!

## ROOT VARIATIONS

Sassafras, licorice, burdock, dandelion, sarsaparilla, and wintergreen are some of the roots traditionally used for making "root beer." You can experiment with adding these to a ginger ale and reducing the amount of ginger while keeping the ratio of water to sugar the same. Licorice and dandelion are frequently available as herbal teas; burdock is generally easy to find at Asian markets. Sassafras can be found in the wild or bought on the Internet.

Note that some components of sassafras have been found to be carcinogenic to laboratory animals in high concentrations; for this reason, and perhaps because sassafras extract is a precursor to some hallucinogenic drugs, the FDA has banned certain sassafras preparations. But unless you plan on drinking gallons of strong sassafras tea per day, sassafras is probably the least of your worries. For instance, all of the following are probably bigger concerns: if eating fried foods (in which carcinogens are formed during the frying process), eating bananas (which are mildly radioactive), or living at high altitudes or traveling on airplanes (where you are exposed to increased levels of radiation due to less atmospheric protection.

# CHAPTER 8

# MEAT AND OTHER FERMENTED FOODS

JUST AS VEGETABLES AND FRUITS can be preserved, so can meats. And just as microbes can assist in preserving vegetables and fruits, so can they assist in preserving meats.

But as much as I encourage experimentation when fermenting vegetables, fruit, and beverages, I do not encourage it when preserving meats. Preserving meats with fermentation is trickier than fermenting vegetables and fruits, for a couple of reasons. First, meats do not naturally attract friendly microbes the way plants do; in fact, they tend to attract noxious ones. Second, meats do not provide as nice a home for friendly microbes: Friendly bacteria and yeasts prefer sugars and starches, abundant in fruits and vegetables but less abundant in meats, which are made up primarily of proteins and fats.

SO WHEN YOU ARE USING fermentation to help preserve meats, some care is essential.

**Follow precise instructions:** It is not a good idea to be casual about ingredients and amounts in recipes. The heavy dose of salt in a particular formula, for instance, may be necessary to lower the amount of moisture in some meat, making it less appealing to toxic bacteria.

**Always use fresh starters:** Any starters or cultures must be fresh to ensure that they will be active and do their job well.

To make meats completely shelf stable, it is generally necessary to (1) dry, heavily salt, and/or smoke them significantly (like jerky, dried sausage, or salt pork); (2) cure them under specific, controlled conditions that are difficult to duplicate in a home kitchen;

(3) use preservative chemicals; or, most frequently, (4) some combination of all of the above. Other options for long-term meat preserving are pickling using vinegar, canning, and, as most of us have done with meats, freezing.

This is not a book about drying, heavy salting, smoking, vinegaring, canning, or freezing; and it is *definitely* not a book about preservative chemicals. If we use none of these, then our options for preserving meats are limited, and we may not be able to preserve meat for a long time—but with fermentation, we can extend their life somewhat, and we can still enjoy the new flavors created by the process.

# CORNED BEEF

Corned beef has nothing to do with corn. In fact, long before European colonizers had crossed the Atlantic Ocean and brought back maize from the Americas, the English word "corn" was used to refer to any kind of grain—in fact, the words "corn" and "grain" share the same root. So "corn" was used to describe anything grain-like, and in the case of corned beef, "corn" referred to the coarse grains of salt used in the preserving process.

When people relied on salt for long-term meat preserving, they had to use a lot of salt—too much for modern tastes. Today, preservative chemicals are often used in place of some of the salt.

Rather than using an unpalatable amount of salt or going the chemical route, the recipe below adds a whey starter to create a colony of friendly bacteria, plus some sugar to feed the starter. Note that the recipe does not preserve for the long term, the way some of the other recipes in this book do; this corned beef should keep in the refrigerator for up to two weeks.

This recipe is based on a recipe by Sally Fallon from her book *Nourishing Traditions*.

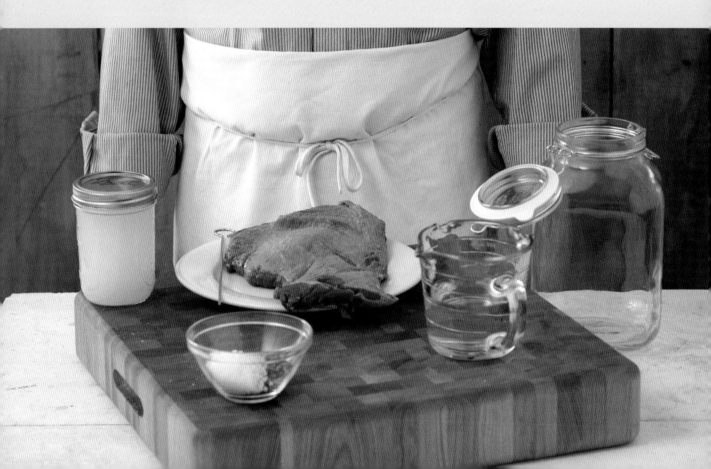

Yield: Approximately 2 pounds (900 g)

Prep time: 20 minutes

Total time: 2 days

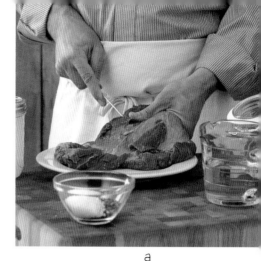

a

## INGREDIENTS

1 beef brisket flat, approximately 2 pounds (900 g)

3 tablespoons (45 g) sea salt (see page 48)

2 tablespoons (25 g) sugar, or caloric sweetener of your choice (rapadura, muscovado, molasses, and brown sugar are good choices)

3 tablespoons (20 g) pickling spice, or whatever spice mix you like

½ cup (125 ml) whey (see page 102)

1 cup (250 ml) nonchlorinated water

## EQUIPMENT

Long, sharp object, such as a skewer, or tines of a meat fork

2 small bowls, with a cover or plastic wrap to cover one of them

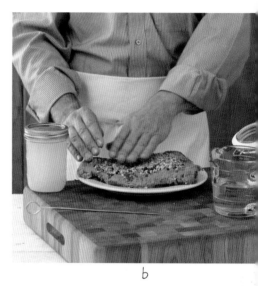

b

## PREPARATION

1   Pierce the brisket many times, quite deeply, with a metal skewer or other long, sharp object (a).

2   Mix the dry seasonings in a bowl and then rub them into the brisket (b). Place the brisket in a bowl or jar.

3   Mix the whey with the water, then pour the mixture over the brisket, making sure that it is completely submerged (c). If you need more liquid, make more brine using 1 cup (250 ml) water, ½ cup (125 ml) whey, and 3 tablespoons (45 g) salt.

4   Cover the bowl with a cover of some sort or close the jar. (If you use plastic wrap, make sure that the plastic is not touching the meat or the liquid.) Allow the meat to sit for a day at room temperature, turning every several hours and making sure that the meat remains submerged. Then refrigerate for at least a day and up to 2 weeks.

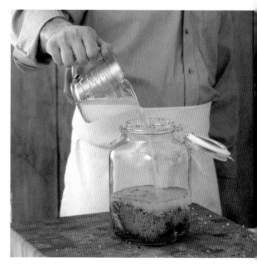

c

## PREPARATION IDEAS FOR CORNED BEEF

------------------------------

**Raw Corned Beef:** Trim away the tough parts of the brisket with a knife. Slice it as thinly as possible, against the grain. Use a deli meat slicing machine if you have one, or else the best slicing knife you have. Enjoy it as part of a cold meat platter or on a sandwich.

**Corned Beef Jerky:** Slice corned beef into 1-inch (2.5 cm)-thick strips, with the grain. Dry it in a 165°F (74°C) oven or in a food dehydrator on a high heat setting. (At lower temperatures, the wrong sorts of microbes might grow too quickly.) When done, it should be dry but pliable, not brittle. Store it in an airtight container and eat it within a week.

**Boiled Corned Beef:** Put the corned beef in a stockpot with a couple of onions, fill with water to cover by at least a few inches, boil it for 30 minutes, then cover and simmer for 3 hours over low heat. If you'd like, add carrots, potatoes, cabbage, and more water to cover, and cook another 30 minutes. Remove the vegetables and plate them. Remove the corned beef, slice it rather thickly, and serve it, with mustard on the side if desired. Use the boiling liquid as a sauce; serve it as a soup later if you like, reducing it first if you want a stronger soup.

**Braised Corned Beef:** Put the corned beef, fat side up, in a large saucepan or enameled casserole with a tight-fitting lid. Choose a braising liquid; light-bodied beer works well. Add your liquid to the cooking vessel until it comes halfway up the sides of the corned beef. Cook, covered, at a bare simmer on the stovetop until the meat is perfectly tender, 2 or 3 or more hours depending on the thickness of the brisket. (Test it with a fork; you should be able to pierce the beef with hardly any resistance.) Remove the beef to a platter and cover it to keep it from drying out. If you like, boil down the braising liquid to desired taste and thickness, and serve it as a sauce. Slice as desired.

**Corned beef sandwiches:**

* Homemade mustard on rye bread

* The Reuben: rye bread, sauerkraut, Swiss cheese, Russian dressing

* The Rachel: brioche, coleslaw, Swiss cheese, Russian dressing

* The Kimchi Reuben: bread, kimchi, Swiss cheese, Russian dressing

* Or, of course, invent your own sandwich that showcases and complements the spiced flavors of corned beef.

The pink or red color of commercial corned beef is due to the use of preservative chemical salts such as sodium nitrite, which may be carcinogenic. Not recommended.

# MORE FERMENTED FOODS

The following section is an extended visual glossary of some other (delicious) fermented foods. I offer you an overview of the fermenting process, but no step-by-step recipes. And because bread is a cultural staple, like wine and beer, there are myriad bread resources available out there for anyone who would like to learn more about bread making.

## DRIED SAUSAGES

The white coating on the outside of some dried sausages is a combination of edible yeasts and molds.

## FERMENTED FISH

Fish, often anchovies, are packed in a barrel with large amounts of salt and left to sit. The fish ferment, and the salt draws the water out of them. The resulting liquid, known as fish sauce, plays a significant role in many cuisines, including those of Southeast and East Asia (where it goes by many names, including *nuoc mam, nam pla, patis,* and *ishiru*). In the West, there is Worcestershire sauce, which typically contains fermented anchovy extract; it may trace its roots back to ancient Greek and Roman cuisines, in which fish sauce was a staple. In Scandinavia, the fish themselves are eaten.

Fermented fish and fish sauce are excellent sources of free amino acids and of vitamin $B_{12}$, although because of their strong flavor and saltiness, they are used sparingly.

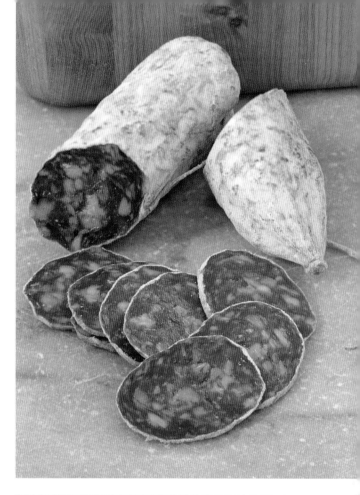

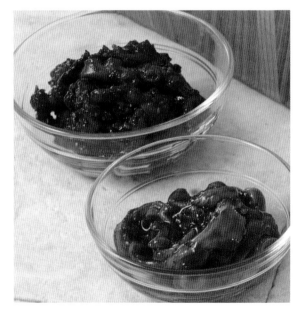

IN KOREA, FERMENTED SQUID AND OCTOPUS ROUTINELY FIND THEIR WAY ONTO THE TABLE AS SIDE DISHES.

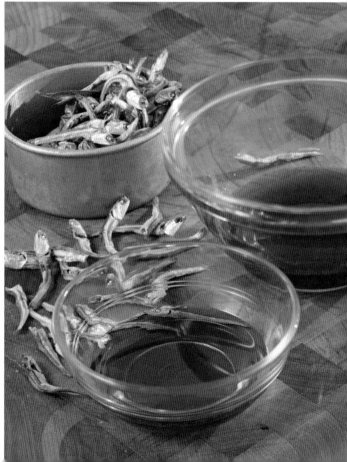

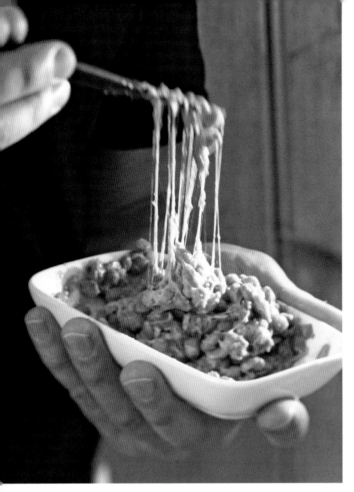

## FERMENTED SOY

**Soy sauce** is probably the most widespread fermented soy food. It is made by fermenting soybeans with a specific type of mold and salt, then pressing out the liquid.

**Tempeh** is another soy ferment made with different types of mold; tempeh is eaten as solid cakes of relatively intact, fermented soybeans.

**Natto** (pictured) is the product of fermenting soy with a particular type of bacteria. Its texture is stringy and slimy, its flavor is strong, and people tend to have strong opinions about it, one way or the other.

**Miso** is a paste resulting from the fermentation of soy via a fungus; it too is strongly flavored, but it is less controversial than its bacterially fermented cousin, natto.

It is worth noting that tofu is not generally a fermented food (although tofu can be fermented after it is made). It is also worth noting that soy should not be eaten in large amounts, because of its potentially negative effects on the human endocrine system. Fermented soy is better than unfermented soy in this regard, but should still be used sparingly.

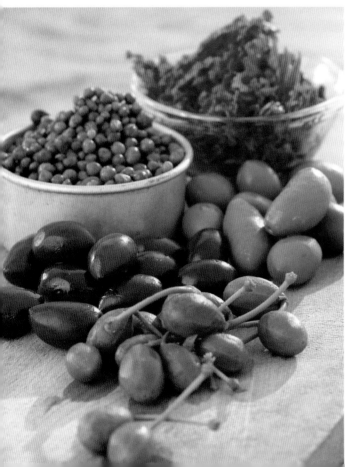

## OLIVES, CAPERS, AND CAPERBERRIES

Capers, caperberries, and many kinds of olives are brined and fermented before we eat them. The fermentation process neutralizes compounds in olives that would otherwise make them unpleasantly bitter. They are staples in Mediterranean cuisine.

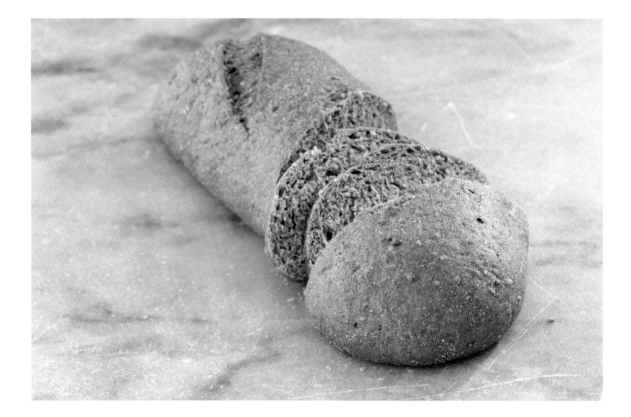

## BREAD

Bread is an iconic food. "Breaking bread" with someone is more than just a physical act; it implies camaraderie and fellowship. And when the Christian Book of Matthew says, "Give us this day our daily bread," it is talking about more than just bread—it is talking about sustenance and continuity.

It may come as no surprise, then—especially if you have been reading this book from the beginning!—that bread is a fermented food.

Fermenting bread requires a starter. You can pull a starter out of thin air (literally) by creating the right conditions for wild yeasts to settle on your dough. A more reliable method is to maintain your own colony of bread starter and use a bit of it to start the fermentation process each time you want to make bread.

Traditional breadmaking involves a long, slow rise, sometimes over a couple of days; modern methods are quicker, use yeast cake or granules bought at the store, and result in bread that is less tasty and less nutritious.

The yeast in the starter ferments some of the flour, generating carbon dioxide and small amounts of alcohol in the process. The carbon dioxide is responsible for the rise of the dough, both before going into the oven and when it first gets in the oven. The alcohol evaporates quickly once the bread is in the oven.

Sadly, the microbes do not survive the baking of the bread. But we can summon them again the next time we need them, and we know that they will come.

# RESOURCES

Some of the resources below are mentioned in this book. This resource list can also be found online at http://RealFoodFermentation.com/resources, where all the items are clickable. The online version of this list will be updated regularly and will continue to grow.

## BOOKS

*Appetite for Change: How the Counterculture Took on the Food Industry* by Warren Belasco
A fascinating documentation of the ongoing culture war surrounding access to food.

*Home Cheese Making* by Ricki Carroll
The reference how-to book by the person who started the modern small-scale cheese-making movement in the United States.

*The Jungle: The Uncensored Original Edition* by Upton Sinclair
A singular document of the horrors of the early industrial meat industry, unexpurgated and as the author intended it to be read.

*The Kimchi Chronicles: Korean Cooking for an American Kitchen* by Maria Vongerichten
A beautiful book that includes a lot of ideas for how to cook with one of our favorite fermented foods.

*Kombucha: Healthy Beverage and Natural Remedy from the Far East* by Günter Frank
A meticulous and thorough book about the "dos" and "don'ts" of making kombucha.

*The Long Emergency: Surviving the End of Oil, Climate Change, and Other Converging Catastrophes of the Twenty-First Century* by James Howard Kunstler
A convincing case for the urgency of the problems facing our world, and why you should learn to make your own food!

*Manifestos on the Future of Food and Seed edited* by Vandana Shiva
A collection of compelling essays on the problems of modern industrial food, and a bold attempt to solve these problems.

*Meat: A Benign Extravagance* by Simon Fairlie
The author makes a meticulously crafted argument that meat production and consumption can be environmentally sound, even advantageous, if done properly.

*Milk: The Surprising Story of Milk Through the Ages* by Anne Mendelson
Everything you never knew you didn't know about milk and dairy, including recipes, in a thoroughly entertaining and lovely book.

*Nourishing Traditions: The Cookbook that Challenges Politically Correct Nutrition and the Diet Dictocrats* by Sally Fallon Morell and Mary G. Enig
The best modern nutrition writing I've come across—followed by a unique description of a wide range of traditional food preparations.

*Nutrition and Physical Degeneration* by Weston A. Price
Dr. Price's detective work uncovers 14 isolated groups of people with exemplary health, and finds and documents commonalities among their diets.

*On Food and Cooking: The Science and Lore of the Kitchen* by Harold McGee
The modern food science reference. Anyone wanting to know about the "why" of food can get this book, and chances are they will find their answers within.

*The Raw Milk Revolution* by David Gumpert
A very engaging window on the current ongoing battles between food regulators and big business on one side and individuals and small farmers on the other over the question of who gets to decide what foods are legal and illegal, written with the pace of a good thriller.

*The Revolution Will Not Be Microwaved: Inside America's Underground Food Movements* by Sandor Katz
Reading this book helped me understand how all the pieces of the food puzzle fit together, and along the way managed to excite and move me more than any book in recent memory—informative, authentic, and passionate.

*Seeds of Deception: Exposing Industry and Government Lies About the Safety of the Genetically Engineered Foods You're Eating* by Jeffrey M. Smith
A provocative look at the increasing evidence that genetically modified foods are a growing disaster.

*ServSafe Coursebook* by Association Solutions National Restaurant Association
This is the United States food industry reference on food safety.

*Silent Spring* by Rachel Carson.
The book that started the modern environmental movement.

*Wild Fermentation: The Flavor, Nutrition, and Craft of Live-Culture Foods* by Sandor Katz
An awesome look at the ancient art of fermentation and its place in the context of our modern existence, including lots of recipes. A must-have for any serious—or even casual—fermenter. The book that put sauerkraut back on the map.

## FILMS

*Farmageddon* (2011)
Kristin Canty sheds light on egregious over reaches by regulatory and law enforcement agencies, creating and imposing unreasonable policies at the expense of farmers and private individuals.

*Food, Inc.* (2008)
Exposes how modern food production feeds the wallets of food industry hegemons at the expense of ordinary, particularly rural, and lower-income people.

*Fresh* (2009)
Exposes some of the problems with our food system, and highlights some of the innovative solutions that people are coming up with.

*The Future of Food* (2004)
Director Deborah Koons Garcia presents a disturbing picture of food technology trends and their impact on society and the environment.

*The World According to Monsanto* (2008)
Filmmaker Marie-Monique Robin tells a disturbing story of collusion between industry and government to control food production at its very root: the farm.

## ORGANIZATIONS

### Weston A. Price Foundation
A fantastic, fast-growing non-profit foundation dedicated to restoring healthy, nutrient-dense, real food to the human diet. Their website is a treasure trove of information about food, diet, and physiology.

### Cornucopia Institute
Seeking economic justice for the family-scale farming community. They provide a plethora of useful information about food—for instance, an egg-buying guide that goes beyond "free-range," "cage-free," and "organic."

### Environmental Working Group
A group focused on environmental toxins. Their "Clean 15/Dirty Dozen" shopper's guide is a great outline of which foods are most important to buy organic.

## OTHER BLOGS AND WEBSITES

### Feed Me Like You Mean It
My blog where I talk about fermentation, real food, raw milk, and where it's all leading, with some recipes.

### Kombucha Fuel
Annabelle Ho's blog follows her extensive experience brewing kombucha, doing live demonstrations, and documenting other kombucha-related events.

### Real Food Media
A network of first-rate bloggers who provide inspiring and informative recipes, stories, and commentary on the subject of real food.

### The Complete Patient
David Gumpert's blog defines the cutting edge of raw milk and food freedom journalism.

## FOOD PRODUCERS, STORES, AND SCHOOLS

### Caldwell Bio Fermentation
A resource for fermentation starters.

### The Cheese School of San Francisco
A great cheese-making school in the heart of San Francisco, California

### Filters Fast
This is where I have bought my water filtration systems.

### Giant Microbes
Stuffed animals, but instead of animals they're microbes. Buy one to make sure you don't raise bacteriophobes.

### The Homebrew Emporium
A great place for brewing-related gear.

### New England Cheesemaking Supply Company
Ricki Carroll's unique cheese-making school, and an online resource for cheese-making supplies.

### Pickl-It
Very reliable fermentation vessels.

### Taza Chocolate
A cutting-edge, small batch chocolate producer.

# ACKNOWLEDGMENTS

There are many people without whom this book would not have happened. I would like to acknowledge as many of them as I can.

Sandor Katz is the grandfather of the modern fermentation revolution. His commitment to fermentation is unparalleled. His fearless humanity is humbling. His writing is brilliant. I feel his presence whenever fermentation is on the table.

If Sandor is the grandfather, then Sally Fallon Morell is the grandmother. Her desire to feed her children healthy food gave birth to an international movement and community, the Weston A. Price Foundation, that is a priceless resource for me and many others, and that has created an ecosystem in which many fermentation and real food businesses have been able to flourish. Among this community, Anne Marie Michaels and the Real Food Media bloggers immediately made me feel at home and have set great examples, and I am very happy to see our real food work continue to germinate.

I am part of a group in Boston called the Sustainable Food Book Club. I would like to thank all the participants in the book club, and in particular Deborah Frieze, with whom I started the club. My thoughts about food matured and solidified as a result of the books we've read and the conversations we've had.

Thank you to Justin Deri who showed me what farmers do, who was eating local food before it was trendy, and who has always been one step ahead of the crowd in matters of food.

Cambridge Culinary Institute, The Institute for Integrative Nutrition, and Learning as Leadership have brought me valuable insights about food, health, and people, each at just the right moment in my life. I would like to thank all who facilitated my learning.

I would like to thank Annabelle Ho, Alex Whitmore, and Corey Beck for their contributions to the book. They are true experts in their respective domains—and they are simply great people. Extra thanks to Alex for introducing me to Quarry Books.

Speaking of which, I would like to thank the team at Quarry Books, without whom there would literally be no book. In particular, Rochelle Bourgault was the ideal editor for me while I was writing the book, providing invaluable brainstorming services and employing just the right amount of stick to help bring the book to fruition.

And of course without my mom, there would be no book. I'd like to thank her for hatching me, cooking with me, eating with me, and for her meticulous proofreading.

Thanks, too, to all the others who have read drafts and provided feedback.

Finally, I'd like to thank my partner Kirstin Falk. She tasted most of my fermentation experiments, even sometimes against her better judgment, and gave me unvarnished feedback. She also put up with my late nights working on the book (or procrastinating and avoiding working on the book). She helped me frame my thinking about the book and its purpose. And she believed in me all along. I am grateful.

# ABOUT THE AUTHOR

Alex Lewin has always loved food, eating, experiments, and puzzles.

After studying math at Harvard and working in the computer industry, he became more and more interested in food and health, in particular the question of what to eat. Buy ten books about diet, and they will tell you ten different things. Why is this?

Cooking school (Cambridge School of Culinary Arts) and nutrition school (Institute for Integrative Nutrition) helped Alex frame general answers: Some of the things that we eat today are simply toxic; different people need different kinds of foods; and, sadly, much of the food and health industry is driven by money and ambition rather than science, wisdom, or compassion.

In order to create a healthier and tastier world, Alex spreads the good news about fermentation, by writing about it here and in his blog, and by teaching fermentation classes and leading workshops. He also serves on the board of the Boston Public Market Association, working to create a year-round indoor market selling local food.

At his day job, Alex writes software, averts disasters, and generally tries to create order out of chaos.

Besides food, health, and computers, his interests include music, all manner of two-wheeled vehicles, cats, and exploring the obscure. He lives in Boston and San Francisco.

To find out more, visit his blog at http://FeedMeLikeYouMeanIt.com. For news and updates about this book, visit http://RealFoodFermentation.com.

# INDEX

# ALSO AVAILABLE FROM QUARRY

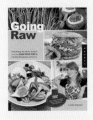

**Going Raw**
978-1-59253-685-6

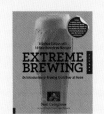

**Extreme Brewing,**
**A Deluxe Edition with**
**14 New Homebrew Recipes**
978-1-59253-802-7

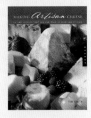

**The Complete**
**Mushroom Hunter**
978-1-59253-615-3

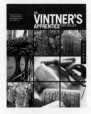

**The Backyard Vintner**
978-1-59253-198-1

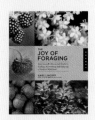

**Making Artisan Cheese**
978-1-59253-197-4

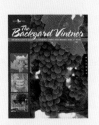

**The Vintner's Apprentice**
978-1-59253-657-3

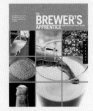

**The Joy of Foraging**
978-1-59253-775-4

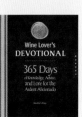

**Wine Lover's Devotional**
978-1-59253-616-0

**The Brewer's Apprentice**
978-1-59253-731-0